THE COMPLETE GUIDE TO
HOLISTIC CAT CARE

BEVERLY MASSACHUSETTS

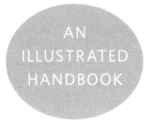

AN ILLUSTRATED HANDBOOK

QUARRY BOOKS

CELESTE YARNALL, PH.D
AND JEAN HOFVE, D.V.M.

Herbs and Supplements • Antiaging Protocols • Raw-Food Preparation

First published in the United States of America by
Quarry Books, a member of
Quayside Publishing Group
100 Cummings Center
Suite 406-L
Beverly, Massachusetts 01915-6101
Telephone: (978) 282-9590
Fax: (978) 283-2742
www.quarrybooks.com

Library of Congress Cataloging-in-Publication Data available

ISBN-13: 978-1-59253-566-8
ISBN-10: 1-59253-566-6

10 9 8 7 6 5 4 3 2 1

Design: bradhamdesign.com
Cover Image: Kevin Mootsey
Back jacket image: © David Muscroft/agefotostock.com
Illustrations: Melanie Powell

Printed in Singapore

A NOTE OF CAUTION

This book is not intended, nor should it be regarded, as veterinary medical advice. Prior to administering any therapeutic course, please consult a doctor of veterinary medicine or a holistic veterinarian. It is their function to diagnose your cat's medical problem and suggest a course of therapy.

Because the authors' approach to cat care is alternative by definition, many of the ideas expressed herein have not been investigated nor approved by any regulatory agencies. National, state, and local laws vary regarding the application or use of these therapies. Accordingly, the reader should not substitute them for treatment by a doctor of veterinary medicine, but rather may use them in conjunction with veterinary care. Always discuss alternative approaches with your doctor of veterinary medicine before embarking upon them. An increasing number of veterinarians are using alternative therapies, and you may wish to consult one or more of them regarding the treatments they offer. Ultimately, you are fully responsible for the health of your feline companion.

The authors and the publisher expressly disclaim responsibility for any adverse reactions or effects resulting from the use of information contained in the following pages.

All photographs, including outdoor shots, were taken under controlled circumstances, and no animals were harmed in any way for these photographs. The authors recommend that cats not be allowed outdoors without a cat-safe harness and lead, or in a cat-safe, secure pen, enclosure, or carrier.

TO ROMEO
the dearest of all and a part of me forever

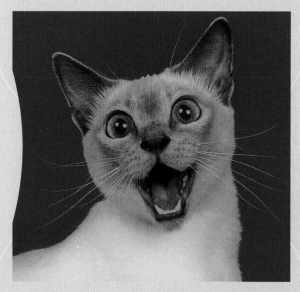

The International Cat Association's Supreme Grand Champion (Alter) Sonham's Romeo of Celestecats, Platinum (Lilac) Point Tonkinese, first generation raw food-fed cat

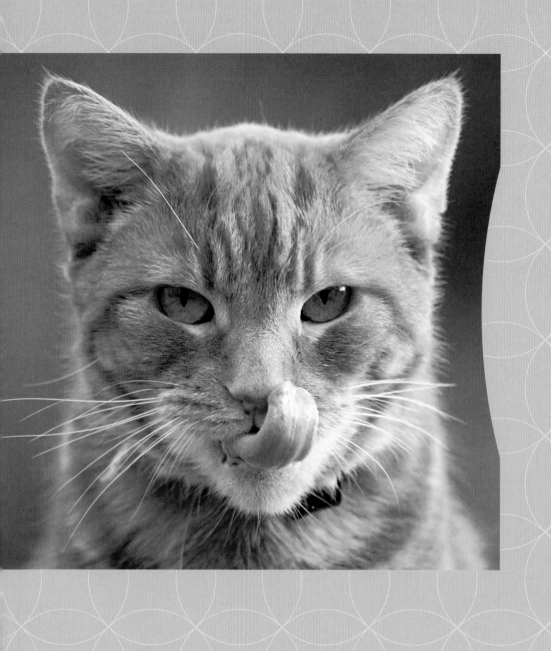

CONTENTS

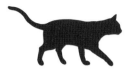

FOREWORD BY JEAN HOFVE, D.V.M.

Now, people who know me will scratch their heads and ask, "Dr. Jean is working with a *breeder*?" I might have asked myself the same thing before I got to know a few folks in the cat fancy and spent some time at cat shows. I applaud Celeste and others who are introducing natural rearing to the world—not just to elite breeders—and showing why it's the best thing for every cat, whether in the show ring or on the sofa.

As we began this project, Celeste came up with a terrific theme: antiaging for cats. Antiaging is the fastest-growing segment of human medicine, and the basic principles that apply to people for living a longer, healthier life apply to our animal companions. They're quite simple in concept: clean environment, good nutrition, satisfying rest, and adequate exercise—in other words, the natural lifestyle we evolved to live. But of course, in the modern world, that's all easier said than done. Even the most remote areas on Earth are no longer pristine, and most of us deal daily with stresses and toxins that make "natural" an impossibly distant goal.

Yet there are certainly ways to combat the forces that are aging us—and our cats—prematurely. Wholesome nutrition is the cornerstone, because how can the body heal if it doesn't have the right groceries? You can give the most expensive, cutting-edge drug, or hold an ancient Mongolian fire healing ritual, or use any other technique you like, but without those fundamental groceries, healing will be impossible.

We'll talk a lot in this book about groceries: the good, the bad, the ugly, and the eeew-get-outta-here. What passes for "complete and balanced nutrition" in the global pet food industry is fairly horrifying. No matter where you live, the best diet is one you make yourself, with wholesome ingredients from a local trustworthy source. In this book, we'll help you do just that, in the best and most healthful way. And don't worry if you're not ready to go whole-hog on our program. Even the smallest step you take on that path will help your cat.

One key topic in this book is alternative veterinary medicine. We'll present you with dozens of options for preventing and treating disease—in particular, the degenerative diseases of aging. It's always best, of course, to work with a holistic veterinarian rather than randomly trying this or that new therapy, and fortunately many excellent holistic vets these days will consult with you by phone.

Some of the modalities (therapies) we discuss will seem pretty far out there. Nevertheless, there are holistic vets who are using these treatments and getting good enough results to keep using them.

My conventional colleagues would no doubt remind us that no matter how many success stories there are, they don't add up to scientific evidence. However, despite the current strong bias toward "evidence-based medicine," the Institute of Medicine, one of the U.S. National Academies of Sciences, carried out an extensive review of mainstream techniques—regular medicines, surgeries, and treatments—and found that up to 20 percent were ineffective and another 21 percent had insufficient evidence to support their use. In other words, the big arguments against alternative medicine can be applied with devastating results to many well-accepted conventional treatments. There is a great deal of science behind modalities such as acupuncture, herbs, nutritional therapy, chiropractic, and even homeopathy.

Conventional medicine and alternative medicine are not mutually exclusive; there are great potential benefits to be gained by combining them. Our purpose in writing about these alternative modalities is to help create a system of "integrative veterinary medicine"—a system that uses the best of conventional and alternative treatments in tailoring an individualized health program for your cat. Certainly, conventional medicine has its place; if your cat has a broken leg, it would be malpractice to prescribe herbs instead of setting the fracture. However, alternative means of pain control, acceleration of healing, and stress management would complement the conventional care.

One vital therapy is attitude—or perhaps, "cattitude." The power of prayer has been scientifically studied and documented, but it's counterproductive to spend 99 percent of the time fretting and worrying and 1 percent of the time praying because in most cases, that 99 percent is going to carry the day. Instead, every time we think about our cats, our health, our future, or any other situation, let's make sure that those thoughts are positive. Remember, whatever you think about that you want, you get; and whatever you think about that you *don't* want, you also get! Wherever we spend the energy currency of our thoughts is what we're buying for the future, so spend it wisely!

INTRODUCTION

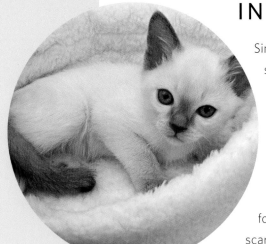

*Cat Fanciers' Association's
Celestecats Bruno Magli Rose,
Platinum Point Tonkinese,
sixth generation raw food-fed kitten*

Since my first book was published in 1995, there have been many scientific advances in both human and veterinary medical care. Many of the subjects I covered—such as acupuncture, chiropractic and natural nutrition and supplements—were considered to be revolutionary concepts; however, today they are accepted therapies and welcomed in the mainstream. In *The Illustrated Guide to Holistic Cat Care* we are again on the cutting edge of medical care. Along with holistic health care modalities for cats, we introduce the concept of antiaging for cats, which is scarcely mentioned in the veterinary vocabulary.

Hopefully, you have already incorporated preventive medicine and antiaging protocols—such as organic foods, exercise, and supplementation—into your own health care regime. In this book, we have collected the best of these preventive protocols, along with antiaging and holistic principles, and adapted what we feel is safe and appropriate for our companion cats. I'm presenting to you ground-breaking material found in the most sophisticated human antiaging regimes. These are not just theories proposed on these pages. They are the very principles and protocols that are the backbone of my eleven-generation championship Tonkinese cat breeding program.

I saw firsthand what this regime produces, generation after generation, and observed the difference between my cats and cats born and raised with commercial pet foods, the overuse of drugs, and annual vaccines. When I raised my first litter in the conventional way, I was so concerned by what I experienced that I began to challenge what I was being told by my vets and breeder mentors. I broke away from those tired methods and launched my own holistic breeding program. Once on the path, I consulted with many experts along the way that included top holistic veterinarians, such as Jean Hofve, D.V.M., who is our voice of authority and resident veterinary expert.

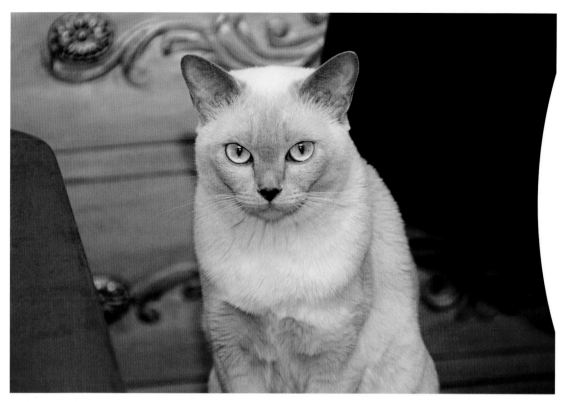

Cat Fanciers' Association's Celestecats Kahlua, Platinum Mink Tonkinese, ninth generation raw food-fed cat

RESPECTING MOTHER NATURE

As a breeder, I read early on that it would take six generations to undo the damage from feeding cooked and processed foods to cats. Each generation of kittens I raised was healthier than the last, with more energy, calmer temperaments, increased muscle tone, and stronger resistance to infections and parasites. With the sixth generation, we saw the end to the teeth and gum problems that virtually all domesticated cats develop by age three.

I called my cats Celestial Cats, "naturally raised" Tonkinese, and I began spreading the word about my unique breeding program at cat shows and other venues.

My agenda was only to help people improve the health of their cats. When my kittens' new guardians incorporated my homemade diet and supplements and implemented our holistic principles, other cat family members' health and wellness also improved. Many of these people even switched to organic and home-prepared foods for themselves.

Veterinarians get very little training on companion animal nutrition in school—a few hours at most, and often taught by someone directly employed or indirectly funded by commercial pet food companies. Most vets' continuing education on the subject comes from their pet food sales reps. This is one area where it will do you well to get yourself educated. You may be able to give your vet an earful!

INTEGRATING HOLISTIC ALTERNATIVES AND CONVENTIONAL VETERINARY MEDICINE

It is not our intent to override your veterinarian's advice, nor do we intend this book to be a substitute for quality veterinary care. We encourage you to become the steward of your cat's health care. Your vet works *for you*. When evaluating a serious problem or disease, allow your vet to run the appropriate tests, but remember that a diagnosis is a well-educated guess. Even when lab work supports that guess, there is still a margin of error. Vets are trained to envision and present the worst case scenario. Your cat's hair ball cough or reaction to clay litter may be diagnosed as asthma; your cat's digestive upset might be labeled inflammatory bowel disease. (I call it inflammatory kibble disease.) However, you have the right—and perhaps the duty—to seek a second opinion from a holistic veterinarian, who might know an effective natural therapy for your cat, or at least be able to offset the side effects of conventional medical procedures.

Inquire about your veterinarian's education, experience, and healing philosophy, and observe how your veterinarian handles and interacts with your cat. Only you can determine who the right practitioner is for you and your cat. Ask as many questions as necessary to fully understand what is involved before you agree to any treatment. Constantly evaluate your cat's response to therapy. Remember, it is a relationship; you're free to change practitioners at any time.

Some holistic veterinarians will work with you by phone. In that case, you will need a local veterinarian to provide diagnostic services, physical exams, and emergency care. (See Resources on page 174 for an online directory of holistic veterinarian practitioners.)

It is critical that you take responsibility for the health of your cat. Don't expect your veterinarian to do that for you. Bring the fresh ideas from this book to your vet. (Better yet, get a copy for him or her.) Do not just accept conventions such as annual vaccinations and the use of dangerous topical pesticides for flea and tick control. These so-called preventative protocols would never be used on people. None of us deserve to be bullied or frightened into doing something we intuitively know is inherently unhealthy and unnecessary.

HOW TO NAVIGATE THIS BOOK

Holistic practitioners offer myriad approaches, many of which are explained in the following chapters.

In chapter 1, "Getting to Know Your Cat," we offer an overview of the history of the cat and introduce modern cats. Chapter 2 teaches the importance of daily exercise and play. We continue on to the dangers of conventional thinking found in chapter 3, covering safe, holistic alternatives to conventional cleaning products in our homes, the basics of nutrition, and when to say no to vaccines and drugs.

In chapter 4, we explore the art of making homemade cat foods and how to properly supplement these meals, in lieu of buying processed foods in cans and bags. In exchange for a little extra time and effort, your cat truly gets the benefits of a natural species-specific diet.

In chapter 5, you will learn about many tried and true holistic modalities, such as homeopathy, herbs, aromatherapy, and flower essences. Chapter 6 explores hands-on healing therapies, such as chiropractic and acupuncture. Chapter 7 introduces new advances in antiaging and energy medicine, which may actually slow down our cats' biological aging process, as well as therapies using light, sound, and other energy modalities.

Chapter 8 is meant to help when you lose one of the ones you love. It was the most difficult to write for me, as I couldn't help remembering those beloved members of my cat family that have crossed the Rainbow Bridge. The end can also be a beginning, as life comes around full circle when you adopt a new kitten or cat.

In our conclusion, we present some ideas of what might just be on the horizon in the area of life extension for our cats. The projected rate of progress for the twenty-first century will be a thousand times greater than what we witnessed in the twentieth century. That is why I pose the question of antiaging for cats. Why not? Let's ask our vets to offer us preventatives and what will be beneficial for our cats' well-being, just like what is breaking through in the world of human antiaging and life-extension. What is presented in this book may slow the clock, and perhaps even reverse one's biological age. Let's all stay healthy long enough to see what science will offer us in the near future.

In the Appendix you will find health reference tools, including an extensive chart of anti-aging supplements and a lighter "dose" of content—an astrology guide for your cat.

We hope you enjoy this journey as much as we have enjoyed bringing it to you. Dr. Jean and I welcome you to the exciting world of holistic and antiaging cat care.

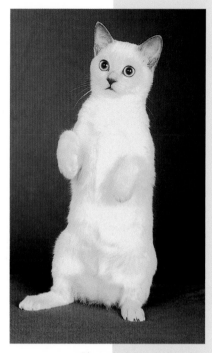

Cat Fanciers' Association's Celestecats Calla Lily, Platinum Mink Tonkinese, fourth generation raw food-fed kitten

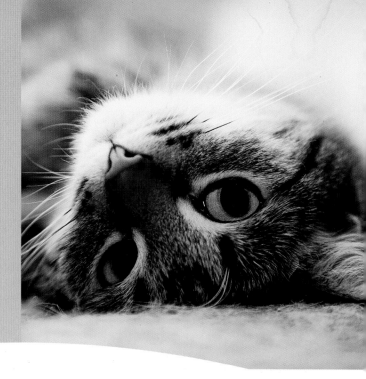

CHAPTER

1

GETTING TO KNOW YOUR CAT

Domestic Shorthair Tabby

As Leonardo da Vinci once said, "The smallest feline is a masterpiece." All cats possess extraordinary sensory abilities, including verbal and non-verbal communication skills, a sophisticated sense of balance and agility, formidable hunting skills, and complex territorial and sexual behaviors.

A BRIEF HISTORY OF THE CAT

The domestic cat remains much the way nature designed its forebears, creatures that lived by hunting and eating other animals. From *Miacis*, over 50 million years ago, (the weasel-like ancestor of all carnivorous animals) and *Dinictis* (the first catlike animal, which appeared ten million years later) descended both the *Viverridae* (civets, genets, mongooses, and meerkats) and the *Felidae* (all modern cats, large and small).

The feline family includes species ranging in size from the tiny 4½ pound (2 kg) African black-footed cat, to the Siberian tiger, a formidable 600 pounds (275 kg) and 10 feet (3 m) long. All modern domesticated breeds belong to the same species, *Felis sylvestris*, and the same subspecies, *Felis sylvestris catus*. Today there are forty-one breeds of cats recognized by the Cat Fanciers' Association, and dozens more are recognized by other international cat associations. All domestic cats are capable of inter-breeding both with one another and, at least theoretically, with wild cats of the *silvestris* species.

It was thought for many years that the Egyptians first domesticated cats some 4,000 years ago. However, French archaeologists have found evidence that our close relationship with cats may have begun even earlier. Carefully interred remains of a human and a cat were found buried with seashells, polished stones, and other decorative artifacts in a 9,500-year-old grave site on the Mediterranean island of Cyprus. This find, from a Neolithic village, predates the Egyptians by 4,000 years or more. The deliberate interment of this animal with a human makes a strong case that cats had a special place in the daily lives and in the afterlives of residents of the village where the remains were found. This particular cat was only eight months old at the time of its death, suggesting that it may have been killed to be buried with its human.

Wild cats were probably drawn to early human settlements, where grain stores attracted rats and mice. Cats were later used specifically to control these pests. This practice gave wild cats a plentiful supply of fresh food, and so began a mutually beneficial relationship between humans and cats.

Some experts believe that the Egyptians may have tamed and bred felines to produce a distinct species by the twentieth or nineteenth century B.C. Cats are frequently represented in Egyptian mythology in the form of the feline goddesses Bastet, Sekhmet, and other deities.

As revered as cats were in ancient Egypt, they were reviled and persecuted in medieval Europe. This era was certainly the Dark Ages for cats, too, but they survived to be prized in modern times as a beloved companion to humans.

LOVING CATS IS ANCIENT HISTORY!

Despite what 9,500-year-old archaeological finds imply, cats are not native to Cyprus. Humans must have introduced cats to their island home along with other farm animals such as pigs, goats, deer, and cattle, which we know they transported by boat—perhaps on a kind of "Noah's Ark" livestock-introduction plan.

Researchers have also stumbled across hints that cats were domesticated even earlier. They have uncovered 10,000-year-old engravings and pottery that depict cats dating to the Neolithic period.

THE MODERN CAT

Many dozens of pedigreed cat breeds have been standardized and registered in Europe and North America. Space will not allow us to talk about each breed in this book, but there are many excellent references on the subject.

Despite the different sizes, shapes, and colors of cats, the needs of our modern domesticated cats are identical to those of their wild cousins. Anatomically and physiologically, the tiger and the tabby are, apart from size, the same. A few thousand years of domestication is not enough time for any significant physiological changes to occur. Modern medicine and processed pet food are too new to cats to have caused changes either.

Other than lions, all cats are antisocial, and domestication has not changed this. Since we are responsible for satisfying our cats' daily physical, mental, social, and emotional needs, duplicating the natural feline diet and lifestyle as closely as we can (within the comfort and safety of our homes) is the best road to health and long life.

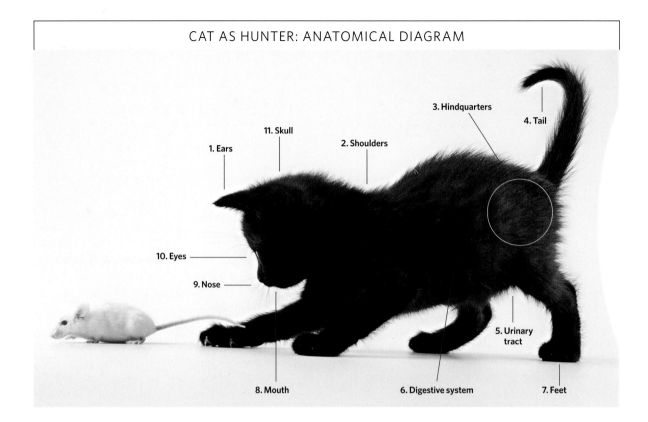

CAT, THE OBLIGATE CARNIVORE

Cats are intended by nature to receive all their nourishment from killing and eating other animals. They have many anatomical and physiological adaptations that make them the perfect hunting machine.

1. A cat's ears are sensitive to extremely high-pitched sounds, including the ultrasonic calls of rodents and insects.

2. A cat's strong shoulder muscles allow for low, slow, stalking movement.

3. A cat has powerful hindquarters that enable him to propel himself up and forward for pouncing on the prey animal.

4. A cat's tail counterbalances quick moves during running and leaping for prey. (Manx cats make up for their lack of tail with their longer hind legs.)

5. A cat's urinary tract pH needs to be an acidic 6.5, which is what a diet of whole mice would produce.

6. A cat's digestive system is designed to handle high-protein meals and does not process carbohydrates very well.

The small intestine lacks brush-border enzymes to convert beta-carotene found in plants to vitamin A. The cat must consume pre-formed vitamin A, which is found in the liver of its prey animal.

The cecum, a part of the large intestine that breaks down fiber, especially in horses, is almost nonexistent in cats. (In humans it is the appendix.)

7. The pads on the bottom of cats' feet are sensitive, thick, and resilient. These pads allow cats to silently stalk their prey. Their claws are curved for gripping and holding their prey. They are also retractable to keep them needle-sharp and in perfect condition. The claws have specialized nerve endings at their bases (identical to those at the base of the whiskers) to allow a precision grip.

8. A cat's tongue is covered with backward-pointing hooks called papillae. The four canine teeth are long and wedge-shaped with pressure-sensitive nerve endings at their bases.

9. A cat's sense of smell is more than ten times as sensitive as a human's.

(10) A cat's vision is keen. It excels in the dim light of dusk and dawn, when prey are most active.

(11) A cat has a thick skull, strong and large to serve as a foundation for the powerful jaw muscles used in catching prey.

THE "ANTISOCIAL" IMMUNE SYSTEM

All cats, except lions, are lone hunters. They are social as kittens, learning life's lessons from mom and tussling with siblings. When they are mature enough, however, they venture out on their own, and they generally remain solitary for the rest of their lives. During estrus (heat or season), these loners come together for mating, then separate. The female gives birth alone, and the male does not participate in raising the young.

Domestic cats have not developed a socialized immune system the way lions have. When you bring a new cat into a multi-pet household, you blend different eco-systems (bacteria and viruses) that tag along from the rescue facility, the breeder's environment, or even your shoes, and the new cat's immune system must contend with an ever-changing ecosystem. (The danger to a new cat comes from other cats, not the parakeet or the German Shepherd Dog.) Without a socialized immune system, a multi-cat scenario can present a problem to the new cat. If possible, plan a period of quarantine for the newcomer, to decompress from the stress of the change of residence, because they are especially vulnerable to a myriad of feline viruses. Therefore, it's important to do everything you can to boost your cat's immune system and limit stress. (See immune-boosting supplements listed in Appendix 1 on page 152.) Do not rely on vaccines alone to protect your kitten or cat. (See chapter 3 for more on this topic.)

A HOLISTIC APPROACH TO CAT CARE

What is holistic health care and how does it relate to your cat? The term "holistic" recognizes that the whole is more than just the sum of its parts. In holistic medicine, the whole being is considered: environment, social and spiritual factors, personality, and emotions, not just the symptomatic parts. Holism, as popularized in the 1960s and 1970s, was a backlash against the Cartesian reductionism—the idea that complex natural phenomena can be explained by reducing them to their constituent parts—that still dominates Western science and medicine today. Philosopher René Descartes, the seventeenth-century mathematician who wrote, "I think, therefore I am," somewhat perversely saw *nonhuman* animals as a mindless, soulless collections of parts, instincts, and reactions that could be taken apart and analyzed and thus understood. This belief led to the use of animals as labor, experimental subjects, clothing, food, and entertainment, with little if any consideration for their feelings.

THE IMPORTANCE OF SPAYING AND NEUTERING

The importance of spaying and neutering cannot be underestimated. Altering our pets makes them far easier for us to live with. We all must do our part to prevent pet overpopulation, as well.

SPAYING FEMALES

Many people do not realize that female cats are perfectly capable of spraying and will urine-mark territory the same way as a male. Spaying the female before her first estrus (heat or season) can prevent this marking behavior. Hormones primarily drive these territorial instincts; female kittens can have their first heat cycle between four and six months of age.

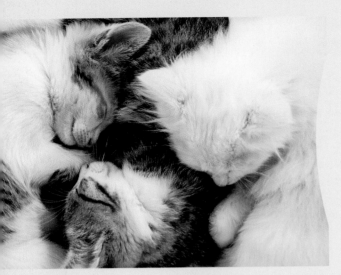

Tabby and White Domestic Shorthair Kittens

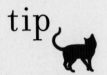

tip

Housekeeping: Keep Your Home Pest-Free

Consider establishing the rule that shoes must be removed when entering your home. Fleas, flea larvae, and life-threatening viruses such as feline panleukopenia (also called feline distemper) can be tracked onto your floors and carpeting. This is especially important when bringing a new kitten or cat home.

A life-threatening condition called pyometra occurs in unspayed females when they come into estrus without being bred. The emergency treatment is most often a very expensive spay. If your cat is not to be a part of a conscientious breeding program, she needs to be spayed no later than six months of age.

During a heat cycle, the female cat does not produce a bloody discharge, like dogs do, unless she has the above-described life-threatening pyometra. She will call for a male suitor nonstop, and writhe in agony for weeks! This is normal behavior for the female cat in estrus. You and your neighbors will experience many sleepless nights because of her incessant "calling" while she is in season.

NEUTERING MALES

When males are not neutered, they spray urine several times per day. Tomcat urine has a very strong and pungent odor. This odor is almost impossible to remove, and the habit is quite difficult to break. They, too, will call loudly to attract females and pace incessantly. An unneutered male cat will escape from your home every chance he gets. The male cat can also be quite aggressive, especially with other male cats, which can lead to fighting, abscesses, and feline AIDS (feline immunodeficiency virus), which is transmitted through bite wounds. This alone is a powerful reason to keep all cats indoors at all times unless on a harness and leash or in a cat-safe play pen, carrier, or enclosure.

The bottom line for intact males and females is that all they think about, besides food, is reproduction. That is what Mother Nature demands of living things, and it is a tremendously strong instinct. However, in our companion cats, it is a distressing and uncomfortable state to be in. Most shelters spay and neuter cats as early as eight weeks of age, because they have no choice but to do so before adoption. Given the option, waiting until they are more mature, at four to six months, works well. Initial studies showed that there were no long-term effects from eight-week spay or neuter, but this is not so clear any more. We especially prefer to wait with males until their urinary tracts are more developed, to prevent later litter box problems and urinary blockage.

The Temptation to Have "Just One Litter"

Many well-meaning folks think it might be fun, interesting, or profitable to breed their cats. However, there is little fun, a lot of hard work, and much peril in breeding cats. Most breeders are thrilled if they can break even; it is not a profitable hobby. It can be dangerous for the male (he can be injured severely by the female); it's very stressful for the female, and complications requiring veterinary care can be expensive as well as lethal.

Others think, "Wouldn't it be good to let the kids see a litter being born?" The answer again is no; there's no guarantee that the kids will be home (or awake) when the birth occurs; instead let the kids watch a video online. (There are many!)

Intentional and accidental pregnancies ("Let's just have the litter and advertise the kittens in a local paper") constitutes "backyard breeding," and this is what fills our shelters with unwanted pets every day, most of which end up being euthanized—even adorable kittens. Mixed breed kittens are not in demand, and the genetics are a wild card.

Please help us reduce the number of cats and kittens that need adoption rather than adding to the problem. As a conscientious breeder, I am trying to leave a legacy that will improve the health of cats for generations to come and undo the damage that irresponsible backyard breeders and kitten mills have caused. There is so much to know and so much to learn that "just having one litter" is a dangerous proposition.

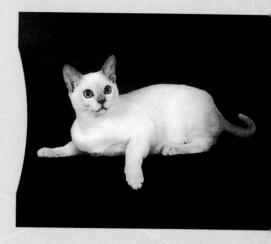

Cat Fanciers' Association's Grand Champion Celestecats Jacques Cartier Rose, Platinum Mink Tonkinese, sixth generation raw food–fed kitten

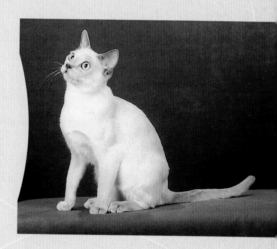

Cat Fanciers' Association's Grand Champion Celestecats American Beauty Rose, Distinguished Merit, Platinum Mink Tonkinese, fifth generation raw food–fed cat

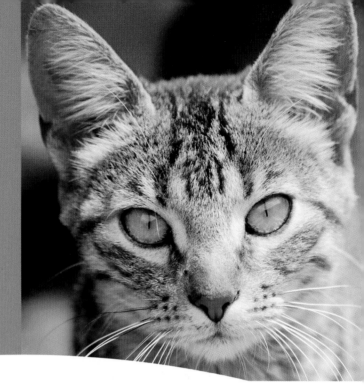

CHAPTER

2

LIVING HARMONIOUSLY WITH YOUR CAT

Domestic Shorthair Tabby

In the following sections, we'll cover some methods of interaction and communication designed to help you deepen your bond with your cat family. If you are just starting out with a brand new addition to your family, either a kitten or adult, this information will help you learn the basics of human-feline interaction as well as deepening and strengthening the bond and relationship with your cat. If you are contemplating adding a cat to your household, knowing what is involved from the holistic point of view can also be beneficial.

BRINGING YOUR NEW KITTEN OR CAT HOME

You've made the decision to expand your family. Whether you've inherited a cat from a family member or friend, brought home a shelter kitty, decided to let in the neighborhood stray, or you've done your homework and have found a reputable and conscientious breeder, the following tips will help make the transition much smoother.

PREPARE A ROOM IN YOUR HOUSE FOR THE NEW ARRIVAL. He's going to need some time to adjust to his new environment—the new sights, sounds, and smells; the new ecosystem of germs; and the new people—so set the room up for an extended stay. You'll need to provide all the basic creature comforts—water bowl, comfortable bed, and litter box. If you are using a spare bedroom or office for your kitty's temporary quarters, make sure you "kitty-proof" it. Just like with small children, put away anything valuable or breakable. Get down on the floor and look around from a "cat's eye view." Cover any bed, sofa, or upholstered chair with a waterproof pad or sheet. Remember, cats are territorial and may, when feeling insecure, mark their territory with urine or feces. If another animal has been in the room and had a little "accident" that you never noticed, a new cat will find it and "refresh" it!

CLEAN AND PREPARE A PET CARRIER FOR TRANSPORTING YOUR NEW CAT HOME. Wash a pet carrier with a solution of 1:32 bleach and water solution (1 ounce [30 ml] bleach to 1 gallon [4 l] of warm water) and rinse thoroughly. Outfit it with something you've worn, such as a T-shirt, so the kitty can start getting used to your scent on the way home. Once you get the kitty home, you might want to leave the carrier in the room for him as an extra haven of security.

WHEN DRIVING HOME, MAKE SURE THE CARRIER IS SECURED WITH A SEATBELT. Also, driving in a car is usually an intense experience for the cat, so keep the music from your radio or CD player soft and soothing; light classical is a good choice, especially Mozart.

GIVE YOUR NEW KITTY AN ADEQUATE ADJUSTMENT/QUARANTINE PERIOD. This should be a minimum of fourteen days and preferably twenty-one. It will allow for mental, emotional, and immune system adaptation. You, of course, will be in the room frequently to love, feed, and bond with your cat. He will become more comfortable and, of extreme importance, get used to his new litter box. You can start to introduce your new kitty slowly to the rest of your home. Expect the introduction period to take weeks, not days. If you get too excited and/or impatient and rush this time, you risk social failure as well as litter box mistakes.

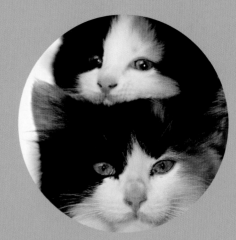

Calico Kittens

One Kitten or Two?

Even though cats are anti-social creatures, they do form bonds with certain other cats. For example, mother cats name their kittens. They have special signals for each one, verbal and nonverbal. Kittens are used to having their family lick their ears and other parts.

In a recent litter of eight, I could easily see teams being formed and friendships made among the siblings. When I pointed out to one of my kitten buyers how closely a brother and sister had bonded, she adopted both of them. Another young woman brought home her "only child," but two days later she returned and acquired another kitten as a pal. I always explain to new kitten parents how important it is for kittens to be adopted in pairs whenever possible. Humans form wonderful friendships with cats, but we'll never *be* cats!

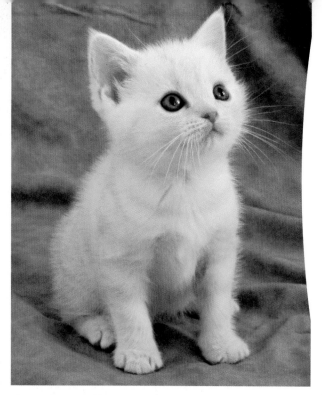

Cream Cameo Tabby American Shorthair Kitten

IF YOU HAVE OTHER PETS, MAKE SURE YOU GIVE THEM PLENTY OF AFFECTION SO THEY DON'T FEEL NEGLECTED, AND MAKE THE INTRODUCTION GRADUALLY. All the animals will be aware of each other by smell first. Feed resident cats and the new cat on opposite sides of the (closed) door to the new cat's room; feed the dog separately due to dogs' natural guarding behaviors surrounding food. (It is never safe to feed dogs and cats together.) Paws may start to reach under the door. Moderate hissing or growling is normal. Gradually crack the door open so the pets can see each other without being able to fight. Occasionally bring some of your resident pets' bedding into the new cat's room, so that the newcomer can become acquainted with the scent. The new cat's bedding can also be introduced to the current residents. Do occasional "territory swaps" by putting the new cat in another part of the house and the resident cats in the new cat's room. Sometimes they become fast friends; sometimes they will annoy but tolerate each other; sometimes the sounds of hissing and yowling will make you wonder if bringing home another cat was the right thing—but don't worry. With cat introductions, some personalities blend and others don't, but in nearly all cases, they can be taught to tolerate each other.

If you're introducing a cat to one or more dogs, keep all dogs leashed at all times to allow the new cat to choose how closely to interact. Never leave any dog and cat together unsupervised (no matter how well they know each other) unless the cat has a good escape route.

LIMIT NEW "SIBLINGS'" TIME TOGETHER IF IT'S NOT GOING WELL INITIALLY. They will decide among them who is going to be "top cat!" Flower essences are excellent aids for introductions and for changes of all kinds. (See "Flower Essences" on page 100.) Helping the cats to socialize through play therapy can also be helpful. (See "Understanding the Importance of Play Therapy" on page 26 and "Play Therapy" on page 29.)

KEEP IT DARK. Let your new cat sleep in a dark room with no light at all. This will help your cat give up any tendency toward nocturnal activities and adjust to your schedule.

COMMUNICATING WITH YOUR CAT

Long before humans had language, we were able to communicate among ourselves and with animals through nonverbal communication. Developing this skill helps us to better interact with and care for our animal companions. Most cat lovers already possess a good working knowledge of feline body language—the subtleties of ear and tail posturing, the dilation of the pupils, and the use of the claws—simply through years of observation. Through nonverbal communication, you can actually begin to see through the cat's eyes and become its voice. Learning the basics is quite easy: Put aside your left brain (the part that uses logic and reason), embrace the right brain (which thinks holistically, using intuition and emotions), and trust the messages you receive. Always send positive images of the desired outcome. For instance, don't send a picture of the cat scratching the sofa unless you want the cat to get the message "OK, now go scratch the sofa!"

Those of us fortunate enough to have been raised with pets "talked" to them and received responses without words. If you remember your own such early experiences, you've probably chalked them up to an extremely active imagination. Or perhaps you once played with a set of twins who told you they each knew what the other was thinking, or you heard your mother say she had "woman's intuition" or "just knew something was wrong." Have you ever had a friend come to mind and then received a phone call from that very person saying, "I was just thinking about you and wanted to say hello"? These are all examples of nonverbal communication.

Try the following at home: Close your eyes. Remember every detail of one of your cats; the feeling of her weight on your lap, her fur, her scratchy tongue licking your hand, those trusting eyes. Visualize her walking toward you or jumping up on your bed. Often, the first time you do this, the cat will be on your lap before you know it, so happy that you've communicated with her in her own language. That is nonverbal communication! Nonverbal communication can be a valuable tool for both lay people as well as holistic practitioners. (See Resources on page 174 for some books on the topic.)

SETTING UP THE LITTER BOX

Cats naturally communicate through their urine, feces, and scent marking. However, when they live with humans, we prefer that they limit these methods of communication! Here are a few tips to help prevent these frustrating problems:

THE MORE THE MERRIER. In multi-cat households, behaviorists recommend one box per cat plus one as the equation for litter box contentment. If you're lucky, your cats will be fine with fewer, but don't count on it.

Cat-Proof Your Home

Items that could be hazardous to toddlers if swallowed are also best kept away from animals, as they too put everything in their mouths. So keep yarn, string, paper clips, pins, needles, rubber bands, and plastic bags in cat-proofed (child-proofed) cupboards or tightly covered containers. Safely recycle or dispose of other potentially harmful materials, such as plastic wrap.

Holiday time presents special hazards to cats. Most experts recommend avoiding Christmas tinsel, including Mylar, and angel hair completely. Keep the poinsettias out of the house. Use common sense!

A cat's tongue has backward-facing barbs. Once a cat starts chewing on string, yarn, thread, fishing line, or similar objects, it will feed itself right down the throat, and the cat will be unable to expel it. The string may become life-threatening as it works its way through the digestive tract; the intestines can bunch up on it and become lacerated. If you're lucky, you'll find the "used" string in the litter box; otherwise, emergency surgery may be necessary. Contact your veterinarian immediately if you know or suspect that your cat has eaten any type of string-like object, especially if the cat is vomiting or not eating. If you see string coming out your cat's backside, *do not pull it out. Seek emergency veterinary care immediately.*

Take care with your choice of houseplants, as some are poisonous to cats. Cats will often nibble on anything new or green or that smells interesting. Most bulbs and many houseplants are toxic to both cats and humans, so be certain to keep them out of reach of children, too!

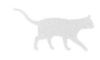

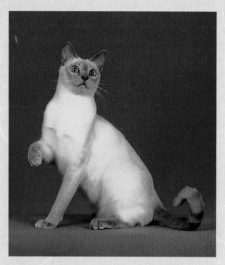

The International Cat Association's Supreme Grand Champion (Alter) Sonham's Romeo of Celestecats, Platinum (Lilac) Point Tonkinese, first generation raw food-fed cat

Ask Your Cat

When I began practicing nonverbal communication with consistency, I wondered if the images I received were fantasy or fact. On one occasion, I brought Romeo (my first Tonkinese kitten) in his carrier to a seminar on nonverbal communication, which was held at an equestrian center. I set up his pup tent (enclosure) and placed his bed and water inside, providing him with his own den. I had to leave him for a few minutes to go across the grounds. In the brief time I was gone, my instructor noticed that Romeo was climbing the sides of his tent and crying. When I returned, I explained that I'd forgotten to tell him I'd be right back, so he felt abandoned and anxious. Even though Romeo was in a tent, the walls were thin and translucent, and nearby there were dogs, horses, and people with cameras. I learned a valuable lesson that day. The incident reminded me that most cats are thinking, "Just tell me what's going on, okay? I worry when you leave me." I also learned how sensitive cats are and how clearly they communicate.

When you leave, it's also important to tell your cat (aloud) when you will return. In a cat's world, when the ones he cares about leave and do not return, it can mean that they have been eaten by predators.

On another occasion, I asked one of my very first cats what made him so frightened when he first came to live with me. He sent me a visual black and white negative image of himself cowering in the back of a carrier, with his sister in front of him, and looking out into an abyss through the door. I remembered picking him up at the baggage claim area at the airport. This beautiful nine-month-old, blue-eyed white Oriental Shorthair male had been locked in his carrier for over eight hours and had wet himself. This experience had made him feel miserable and untrusting of people. He then showed me a beautiful color picture of himself playing with a feather in my bedroom, so I knew he wanted to change the subject. I promised him he'd never have to fly anywhere again.

PLACE LITTER BOXES IN CAT FRIENDLY LOCATIONS. Lining up a row of litter boxes in the basement probably won't cut it. Place a box on every level of the home, especially for older, potentially arthritic cats. Cats don't prefer privacy like we do; in fact, they'd rather have a good view all around so they can see any enemies approaching. Litter boxes in corners or closets may not get used. However, some cats and kittens have become accustomed to them and may prefer to keep it this way. Although privacy is not essential, quiet is. The first time the dryer buzzer goes off while the cat is "doing its business" may be the last time that laundry room box is used.

KEEP IT CLEAN. Cats are fastidious about their hygiene, and a dirty litter box is a turn-off to them. Empty litter boxes daily and wash them in hot soapy water at least weekly or whenever fecal matter clings to the box. Add one drop of lavender essential oil to your organic liquid soap for a pleasant and calming litter box environment, or purchase organic lavender liquid soap. (Do not use products containing ammonia or pine oils while living with cats. Ammonia is a component of cat urine; if you use it in your home, the cat is likely to "refresh" the odor as it fades. Pine oil is both aversive and toxic to cats.)

CHOOSE THE BOX WITH CARE. Some cats don't like boxes with hoods or lids, but many are fine with them. However, since "out of sight is out of mind," if you have trouble remembering to maintain a hooded box, take the lid off. Most holistic practitioners and breeders do not recommend using mechanical, self-cleaning litter boxes as they have a mixed record, especially since clay litter must be used in order for them to run properly.

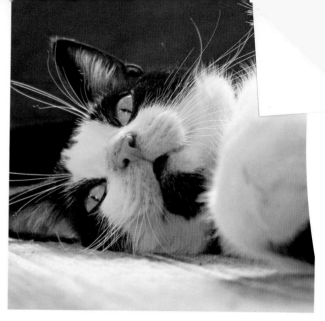

Black and White Domestic Shorthair Bicolor Kitten

CHOOSE RESPONSIBLE, NONTOXIC LITTER. Clay and clumping clay litters are the most common litters, but they're also the most problematic. Litters that contain sodium bentonite clay can be dangerous. Cats lick off and swallow anything that collects on their paws or fur. If young kittens or elderly cats with digestive problems ingest clumping litter, it can cause a blockage in their intestines. The dust from clay litter has been linked to respiratory problems and even asthma. The ideal litter is soft on the paws, not dusty, fragrance-free, easy to manage, and made from a renewable resource. We recommend litter made from corn and wheat, kiln-dried wood shavings or pellets, or non-pine wood pellets (See "Cat Litter" in Resources on page 174 for some suppliers of cat litters.) One way to help your cat adjust to the new litter is to mix the new litter with the old (50–50) and add organic catnip (*Nepeta cataria*) to the box. A small amount of catnip, well-mixed into the litter, encourages digging, which stimulates box use. Reduce the amount of the old litter as your cat uses the new mixture willingly.

NOTE: Litter box problems can be a sign of ill health. Be sure to get your cat checked by the vet before you assume any problem is behavioral.

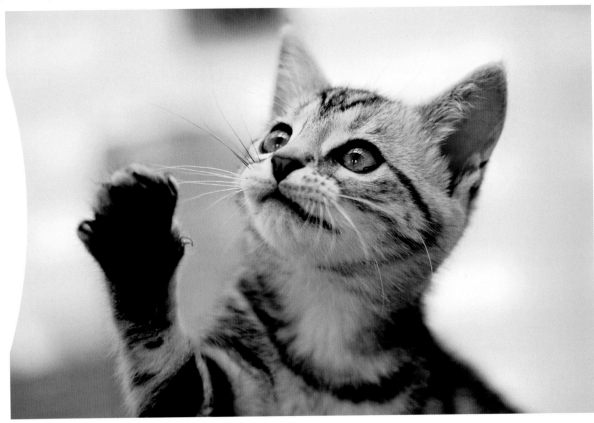

Domestic Shorthair Silver Tabby

UNDERSTANDING THE IMPORTANCE OF PLAY

To enhance the life of your cat, you must understand his needs. In chapter 4, you'll learn about your cat's nutritional needs and how to feed a species-specific diet that provides domesticated cats with everything they need to thrive. However, when we're providing their food, it's missing an important component: the intensity of the hunt and the thrill of capturing the prey. What can we provide as a reasonable substitute for hunting and killing their own food?

Interactive play gives cats exercise and stimulation just like they'd get if they hunted for their dinner. Making time to play with your cat daily, ideally before meals, is essential.

If you have more than one cat, you've likely been an eyewitness to the shenanigans that compatible cat companions get into when left to their own devices. They get their exercise this way, improving their circulation and working up their appetites. Mischief usually starts around dusk, since this is wake-up time for our nocturnal pals. The cats have napped, and they're hungry, so the chase begins. It's mock hunting, a release of pent-up hunting energies. This behavior begins with kittens as young as three to four weeks of age. This exercise is how they explore their world, develop their minds and muscles, and learn how to be cats.

PLAYING GENTLY WITH KITTENS AND CATS

It's tempting to play rough with a kitten, flipping him over and rubbing his little belly, and laughing as, inevitably, the kitten flattens his ears and bites, or rakes the "enemy" with his back feet. While this is cute when a kitten is little, it's much less adorable when the adult cat is armed with powerful claws and razor sharp fangs! For kittens, roughhousing is not play; it's practice for defending their territories and for hunting and catching their prey. Hands are for loving and grooming—never for biting or scratching. It's best not to start, but if your kitten (or cat) has gotten into this bad habit, it needs to be broken. All members of the family need to treat cats and kittens gently. If the cat bites or swats at your hands or feet, just relax and let your limb go limp. It's only interesting while it's moving; when you hold still, the cat will lose interest and walk away. If he doesn't, you'll definitely know better the next time.

Parents always need to supervise young children with cats and kittens. Set a good example for safe, gentle, play sessions. Remember a kitten is not your child's toy; it's a living being. There is nothing better for your child than to grow up with a cat; it will help prevent childhood allergies and build the child's immune system, but the child has to be good for the cat, as well, and that responsibility lies with you, the parent.

NOTE OF CAUTION: Always seek prompt medical attention for bite or puncture wounds.

TRAINING AS PLAY

Cats can be taught to walk on leashes, come when called, fetch and retrieve balls, and jump into your arms when asked. If you think your cat can't learn some tricks, this limitation is coming from you, not the cat. Remember what we learned in nonverbal communication: Project the positive image and the result you hope to attain. Learning to train your cat takes patience, but it offers a wonderful way to bond with your cat or kitten.

YOUR CAT'S AGE IN HUMAN YEARS

AGE OF CAT	AGE OF HUMAN
1 year	15 years
2	24
3	28
4	32
5	36
6	40
7	44
8	48
9	52
10	56
11	60
12	64
13	68
14	72
15	76
16	80
17	84
18	88
19	92
20	96

You've likely heard that a calendar year in a dog's life is equal to seven human years, but this formula isn't accurate for dogs, and certainly not for cats. A two-year-old cat is fully developed and mature, but a fourteen-year-old human isn't. And twenty-year-old cats are not uncommon, but how many 140-year-old humans do you know? The following chart will help you more accurately calculate your cat's age in human terms.

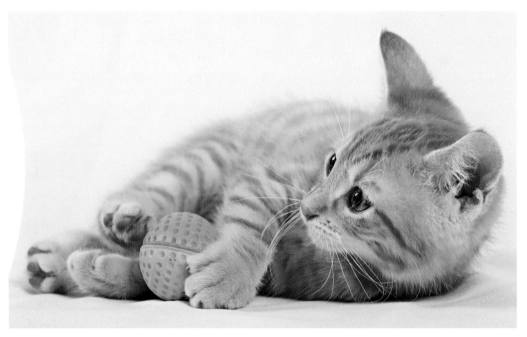

"Marmalade" (red) Domestic Shorthair Kitten

TOYS AND ACCESSORIES

Toys can be as simple as little bits of paper rolled up and tossed for a game of fetch. Watch out because your cat may raid your wastebaskets while you're not around, dumping the contents all over the floor! Ping-Pong balls are great fun, too.

HERE ARE SOME GREAT TOYS AND ACCESSORIES TO CONSIDER.

CATNIP (*Nepeta cataria*) and catnip-filled toys are great fun to introduce to your play area. Put some on the scratching post or cat scratching pads. The scent lasts about a week. Catnip contains the chemical *nepetalactone*, which produces a behavior that closely resembles that of a female in heat, though it doesn't have sexual side effects. Nepetalactone is a hallucinogen, inducing pleasurable sensations and stimulating playful behavior. Response to catnip is genetic; about a third of cats don't react at all. It also doesn't cause any reaction until about six months of age. Responsive cats will sniff it, roll in it, and eat it, and that's all just fine!

Experiment carefully with your cats and catnip, and supervise the ensuing activities, as some cats may respond aggressively. You can also grow fresh catnip. Cats love shredding the little catnip plants. Be sure you grow your catnip organically. Be careful about placement, as many cats will grab the plant and end up dragging the pot all over the carpet.

Never give catnip before a veterinary visit or other potentially stressful event, due to its unpredictable effects in these situations. At cat shows, I often use catnip to amuse my cats, as well as to distract from the smell of the other cats.

CARDBOARD BOXES AND PAPER BAGS (WITHOUT HANDLES) become great hiding places. You can join the fun by instigating a game of hide-and-seek, making little squeaking noises and scratching on the outside of the box or bag, and pouncing from behind walls, doors, or furniture. Think like a cat and have fun!

CAT TREES are essential. It's important for cats to have their own furnishings. A tall, sturdy cat tree is essential, as cats need to climb vertically to develop their full strength. If you don't provide this type of feline jungle gym, your drapes could become the "forest" instead.

Many people notice how active their cats become just before bedtime. While we, their favorite toys, were away at work all day, the cats slept, and now they've got lots of pent up energy to vent. This is another great reason to have more than one cat in your house. They play and cuddle with each other all day while you're gone, and then sleep peacefully through the night. They may also be trying to tell you that it's time for bed and to please turn the TV off as well as the lights, and prepare for bedtime.

PLAY THERAPY

Play therapy is a specific type of structured play done with an interactive fishing pole-type toy on a schedule. Through play therapy, we can harness the cat's natural hunting instinct and use it in a beneficial way. For instance, in multi-cat homes, bullies can be praised for chasing the toy, which is acceptable prey. Shy cats get their confidence boosted by "successful" hunts. Cats that wake their people at all hours can be retrained to sleep when we do by having a play therapy session before bedtime.

Play therapy also creates an immense increase in the guardian-cat bond over time. Your cat will appreciate the difference between nightly sessions of playing with a wand toy and getting praised by you over the furry mice that he or she bats at for two minutes and then loses under the fridge.

Training Sessions

I try to make my cat training sessions fun. I'm paying attention exclusively to the cats, and they love this quality time. My first Tonkinese kitten, Romeo, used to bring me his little ball with the bell for me to throw. He'd repeat this as many as twenty times. If I wasn't available, he'd play by himself or organize a team sport akin to soccer. If the ball got stuck somewhere, he'd call me to rescue it. He'd also practice his dexterity by passing the ball back and forth between his front paws like a soccer player. Some of my other cats throw their toys into the air and pounce on them, then shred them.

Kitty "aerobic classes" are a favorite. I bring out my collection of fishing pole toys. You can make your own by tying any toy or feather to a length of monofilament line (single-strand nylon bead-stringing or fishing line) and attaching it to a stick. Flick it through the air or drag it across the floor. Cats respond to horizontal movements, as this is the way mice scurry when fleeing from them. After play sessions, secure toys with strings and lines safely out of reach, as these toys are interactive and require *you* to be attached to the other end of the toy; otherwise the strings can be chewed and become hazardous. (See "Behavior and Training" in Resources on page 174.)

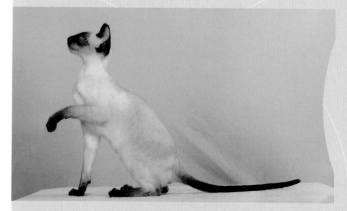

Cat Fanciers' Association's Celestecats Tiffany, Seal Point Oriental Shorthair, second generation raw food-fed cat

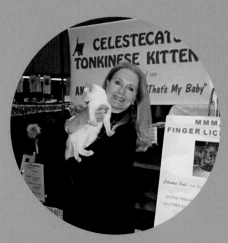

The author, Celeste Yarnall, holding a Platinum Mink Tonkinese cat at a cat show

Come to a Cat Show

I like to invite my cat-loving friends to come see us at one of our Cat Fanciers' Association cat shows, if there's one nearby. You'll find vendors selling an incredible array of cat fun and games, including feline tarot cards for us to tell our cat companion's future!

CAT AGILITY

When we think of agility competitions, we usually think of dogs. Dog agility was loosely modeled on equestrian jumping competitions; it debuted as spectator entertainment at the 1979 Crufts Dog Show in London. Since then, it has become the most rapidly growing dog sport in Western Europe and North America. The International Cat Agility Tournaments (ICAT) has created a similar cat competition where cats display their coordination, speed, and grace of movement in negotiating an agility course.

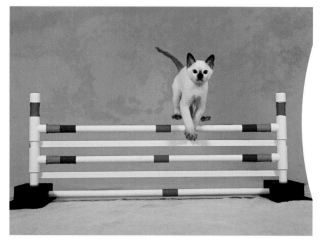

Tonkinese kittens demonstrating cat agility

Abyssinians, Tonkinese, Siamese, and Cornish Rexes are especially suited for cat agility, but any cat can take part. You can most often find cat agility at cat shows, but it can take place anywhere. The course is completely enclosed by high portable fencing. Cat agility is a wonderful way to deepen the bond with our cats. Both pedigreed show cats and household pets can perform, so it is very democratic and certainly not a beauty contest! As the handler trains and guides the cat throughout the course, you see a great relationship between handler and cat. Everyone involved with cat agility hopes to see it become as popular for cats as it is with dogs. It's great to see everyone watching the cats and sharing the handlers' enthusiasm as they race around the course. The cats seem to love it, too.

If your cat is friendly, outgoing, loves to play chase or fetch, and is in good physical condition, you might have an agility star in the making. Here is a checklist to consider:

SELF-CONFIDENCE: Does your cat handle new situations easily, enjoy investigating new things, and find new people interesting? Does your cat love jumping, climbing, and interacting with others? Shyness may limit her competitive ability.

MOTIVATION: Cats love to play, but food is a primary training tool and motivator. You can start by running your cat around the house with a fishing pole-type toy. If she does something well, praise and reward with a tidbit of raw meat. (Cut off a few bits of steak and place

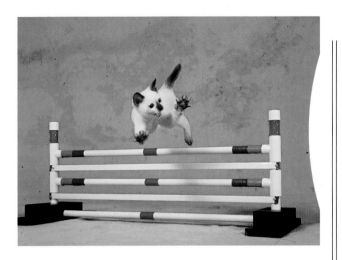

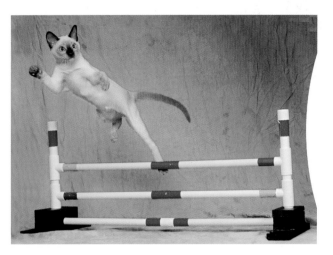

them in a plastic bag before you cook it for your dinner.) Praise and lots of love keep a cat focused.

ATHLETIC ABILITY: Cats need good overall health provided by proper nutrition and exercise. It's a good idea to have your vet check for structural issues (such as hip dysplasia) that would interfere with your cat's ability to run or negotiate obstacles.

TRAINING: Some agility enthusiasts recommend the applied operant conditioning method, which simply means reinforcing a particular response or behavior and/or clicker training. The cat associates the click with getting a reward for a job well done. If your cat makes mistakes, just ignore them and concentrate on rewarding and praising for what is done correctly. Lure her over, under, and through obstacles with a fishing pole toy and your voice. It will always be the cat having the most fun who will do the best.

AGE: The ICAT agility competition is for cats eight months of age and older. Kittens four to eight months old may practice on the basic level course but can not compete.

The Cat Fanciers' Association (CFA) organizes cat agility competitions for CFA sanctioned cat shows, as well as agility enthusiasts. (See Resources, page 174, for more information on how to train and participate in cat agility.)

CAT TRAINING

In the past few years, two training methods, clicker and operant behavior (stimulus-response), have taken the feline world by storm. Once it was thought that cats were too aloof, independent, or stubborn to be trained to do much of anything. It's true that cats aren't dogs. They don't really care if they please us, but they will do something readily—and do it predictably—if it serves them well. Usually by using food as proper motivation, cats can learn to do many of the same basic and advanced tricks as dogs. Operant conditioning works on any species with a nervous system, including chickens, dolphins, humans, and worms. Learning tricks could work well for those cat folks who complain that their companions get bored easily, or can't concentrate through a whole play session.

However you choose to interact with your cat, be sure to include lots of love in your sessions. This is the magical ingredient in all holistic therapies. As children, we loved to play. Who's to tell us we can't still be children with our cats? They won't tell anyone!

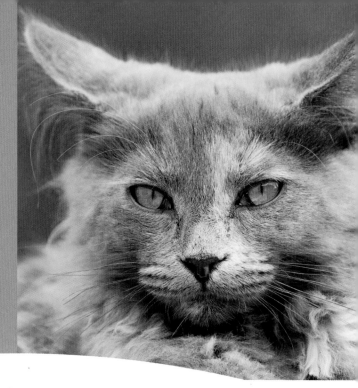

CHAPTER 3

THE DANGERS OF CONVENTIONAL THINKING

Blue Cream Domestic Longhair

There's so much we do to our cats that is accepted and mediocre—so much so that few ever challenge it. But some of these habits have turned out to be quite harmful for our cats. We'll turn some of these notions on their proverbial ears in this chapter as we examine the dangers of conventional thinking.

VACCINATION

Though vaccination has become a highly controversial subject, people who challenge the concept are sometimes treated as if they were against apple pie and motherhood. But, the way vaccines are typically used today, they are extremely dangerous—potentially one of the most harmful things we could do to our animals.

We vaccinate because we're afraid our animals will contract certain diseases. We've accepted annual vaccines without considering where that recommendation came from and what it really means. Most veterinarians recommend cats receive a combination vaccine against panleukopenia (feline distemper), *calicivirus*, and rhinotracheitis (upper respiratory infections). Many also encourage injections for *Chlamydia*, feline leukemia (FeLV), feline immunodeficiency virus (FIV or feline AIDS), feline infectious peritonitis (FIP), and even ringworm. These vaccines are typically repeated every year for the cat's whole life, despite overwhelming scientific evidence that they are unnecessary.

Since the vast majority of vaccines are unnecessary and even unsafe, more and more people are not getting their animals vaccinated at all. However, recent outbreaks of panleukopenia in cats are of great concern. *No* vaccines can be just as dangerous as too many vaccines; the basic kitten shots (panleukopenia and rabies) are still recommended.

Ron Schultz, Ph.D., professor and chair of the department of pathobiological sciences at the University of Wisconsin School of Veterinary Medicine, and Tom R. Phillips, D.V.M., Ph.D., wrote in *Kirk's Current Veterinary Therapy XI* (a book even conventional veterinarians most likely have on the shelf) that:

"A practice that was started many years ago and that lacks scientific validity or verification is annual revaccinations. Almost without exception there is no immunologic requirement for annual revaccination. Immunity to viruses persists for years or for the life of the animal. Successful vaccination to most bacterial pathogens produces an immunologic memory that remains for years allowing an animal to develop a protective anamnestic (secondary) response when exposed to virulent organisms. Only the immune response to toxins requires boosters (e.g., tetanus toxin booster, in humans, is recommended once every seven to ten years), and no toxin vaccines are currently used for dogs or cats. Furthermore, revaccination with most viral vaccines fails to stimulate an anamnestic (secondary) response as a result of interference by existing antibody (similar to maternal antibody interference). The practice of annual vaccination in our opinion should be considered of questionable efficacy unless it is used as a mechanism to provide an annual physical examination or is required by law."

In plain English, this means that the authors believe there is no valid scientific reason to vaccinate pets every year. That practice, instead, emerged as a default judgment between the pharmaceutical companies making the vaccines, and the veterinarians. The vets wanted to get their patients in once a year for a check-up, and the vaccine makers wanted to sell more vaccines. Tying the annual physical to vaccines was a stroke of genius. It simplified life for veterinarians, who now only had to say "We'll see Fluffy next year for his shots" and send a postcard, and it made boatloads of money for the drug companies. When this "suggestion" was added to vaccine

Caution: Overvaccination

Many breeders routinely give vaccines beginning very early and repeating every two weeks. This is a terrible stress on the developing immune system and cause of potential future problems. Ask the person you're getting a kitten or cat from whether it has had any illnesses or medications and what vaccines have been given so you can be sure not to overvaccinate in the future. (It's unnecessary to vaccinate a cat that has already survived panleukopenia because it has a lifetime immunity).

labels, it added an air of "requirement" and ensured that the system would continue to make everyone happy. At the time, vaccines were considered benign—harmless—so this lucrative state of affairs went unquestioned until the late 1980s, when vaccines began to be linked to injection-site cancers in cats.

Today, it is known that vaccines are not so harmless, and they are now considered a medical procedure like any other, with both risks and benefits. In order to realistically assess the situation and make wise decisions for our cats, we need to examine four aspects of vaccination: Are vaccines safe, are vaccines effective, are vaccines necessary, and are there alternatives to vaccines?

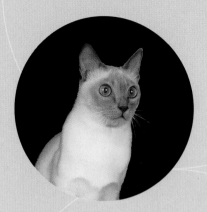

The International Cat Association's Supreme Grand Champion (Alter) Sonham's Romeo of Celestecats, Platinum (Lilac) Point Tonkinese, first generation raw food–fed cat

Romeo Teaches Me a Lesson the Hard Way!

My own Romeo had an upper respiratory infection before I adopted him, and he needed antibiotics before he could come home with me. Thereafter, he developed symptoms of an upper respiratory infection after every vaccination my veterinarian gave him. (This was before I knew about the potential for side effects from vaccines.) It took two weeks of antibiotics before the symptoms seemed to disappear. The second to last time Romeo was vaccinated, he ran a 105°F (40.6°C) fever and was almost comatose four hours after receiving the shot. I helped him by giving him fluids and syringe feeding him broth for days. The next year the veterinarian insisted on vaccinating him again, giving him a dose of an antihistamine first, thinking he was simply allergic to the adjuvant. Four hours later he was running a fever of 105.5°F (40.9°C) and staring into space. Once again I rushed him to the emergency hospital, where he was given steroids and fluids, and I was given strict instructions from the emergency veterinarian never to vaccinate him again!

ARE VACCINES SAFE?

Conventional veterinarians consider a symptom or condition to be an adverse reaction only if it occurs within seventy-two hours of vaccination. Acute reactions are uncommon, but they can be extremely serious, and they can have long-lasting effects.

Holistic veterinarians agree that symptoms of vaccine-induced diseases can occur any time during the life of our cats. In addition, the following known long-term risks are associated with one or more feline vaccines.

AUTOANTIBODIES

Antibodies, blood proteins that attack and destroy invading organisms, are the goal of vaccination. We want the body to produce antibodies against the disease being vaccinated against. However, the vaccine manufacturing process contains some quirks that cause the body to make antibodies to a wide variety of components in the vaccine.

Most vaccines are produced through a culture medium such as eggs, blood serum, or certain types of cells. The organisms are grown in these nutritious cultures, and then filtered for manufacture into vaccines. While the filters are small enough to keep out whole cells, both intended viruses and a variety of unintended loose proteins will end up in the final product. When injected, the animal's body then makes antibodies to many of the proteins as well as the virus itself. Studies at Purdue University showed that canine vaccines grown in calf serum caused antibodies to be made to many calf proteins, including red blood cells, thyroid, DNA, and connective tissue proteins. Unfortunately, calf proteins are so similar to dog proteins that the antibodies react to the puppies' own tissue as well. This is an autoimmune reaction. Every vaccinated puppy developed multiple autoantibodies, and every additional booster produced even more autoantibodies. Because the puppies in the

Purdue study were euthanized at twenty-two weeks of age, it is unknown if these autoantibodies would lead to disease, but logic suggests it is likely. In other words, because proteins are similar among many animals, antibodies to proteins in the vaccines can cause an autoimmune reaction. The immune system starts attacking the body's own organs and tissues.

FELINE CHRONIC RENAL FAILURE

The common feline panleukopenia virus is grown in a culture of feline kidney cells. Recent work at Colorado State University showed that most kittens developed autoantibodies to their own kidney tissues after being vaccinated for panleukopenia. When autoantibodies react with body tissue, the result is inflammation. Each booster vaccine creates even more antibodies—and more inflammation. Chronic low-grade inflammation is the primary cause of feline chronic renal failure (CRF), which is almost guaranteed to develop in older cats. The authors of the study suggest (but did not prove) a causal relationship between the panleukopenia vaccine and the development of CRF.

An auto-immune reaction to kidney proteins injected with the vaccine can cause the cat's immune system to attack its own kidneys. The chronic low-grade inflammation generated by this vaccine reaction—compounded every time the cat receives a booster—is a likely contributor to the development of CRF. Annual boosters for feline panleukopenia are totally unnecessary because the immunity produced by the initial kitten vaccine is very long lasting, and adult cats are naturally resistant.

VACCINE-ASSOCIATED SARCOMAS

Malignant, fatal tumors called fibrosarcomas can be caused by some vaccines in cats. This cancer occurs in the connective tissue. The two vaccines currently implicated are rabies and feline leukemia. A third will undoubtedly be joining the list—the feline AIDS (FIV) vaccine. These three products are all killed vaccines made with adjuvants (substances that increase the immune response). Unfortunately, in cats, this additional response includes inflammation that can lead to the formation of cancer. Even worse, every additional vaccine—indeed, some researchers suggest that every additional injection of any kind (antibiotics, steroids, insulin, sedatives, fluids, etc.)—may significantly increase the risk of developing cancer, particularly if the injections are given in the same place. At least one vaccine maker has recognized this risk and now makes several effective vaccines that do not contain adjuvants, using advanced recombinant technology.

When vaccines were given between the shoulder blades, these cancers were inoperable and fatal because they would grow into the spine, ribcage, and chest. This became such a serious problem that it is now recommended to give the rabies vaccine in the right hind leg, and leukemia in the left hind leg—so that when a tumor does develop, the whole leg can be amputated and thus the cat's life can be saved.

The rabies vaccine is required by law for most animals in most jurisdictions because it is a public health hazard. Therefore, it is important from a legal standpoint to follow your jurisdiction's regulations concerning rabies vaccines for your pets. Killed rabies vaccines are labeled for either one or three years; but the vaccine in the bottle is exactly the same in both cases. The label itself is the only difference. Request that your cat receive the three-year vaccine, only once every three years. Better yet, consider a nonadjuvanted vaccine. If your vet clinic does not carry it, ask if they will order it, or try to find one who does.

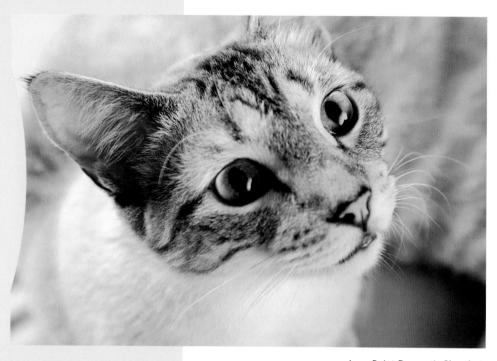

Lynx Point Domestic Shorthair

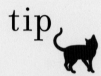

tip

Homeopathic Remedy After Vaccinating

Following a rabies vaccine, give the homeopathic remedy Lyssin 30C or Thuja 30C to help prevent adverse reactions. (See chapter 5 for more information on homeopathy.) Work with your holistic practitioner to minimize health problems that can arise from vaccines.

VACCINOSIS

In homeopathic medicine (explained in Chapter 5), vaccination is considered to cause a chronic condition with multiple symptoms, called vaccinosis. When faced with these symptoms, you may not even see it as a sign of illness. Vaccinosis symptoms include laziness, finickyness, poor grooming habits, hairballs, bladder and kidney problems, chronic vomiting or diarrhea, chronic or recurrent upper respiratory infections, increased or displaced sexual behavior, aggression, destructiveness, wool-sucking, pica (eating indigestible items), seizures, excessive licking, hot spots, and over-grooming. The vaccinosis condition can be inherited as well. Each generation will become more and more ill, unless reversed by nutrition and holistic therapies.

ARE VACCINES EFFECTIVE?

In the history of human vaccines, the numbers clearly show that in every case, the disease itself was already on the decline when the vaccine was introduced. Most vaccines were scarcely a blip on the radar, not affecting the natural decline of the disease at all. In a few unfortunate cases such as polio, the disease actually increased after vaccinations began.

For example, when people contract measles, their overall immune system is strengthened in response to the mild challenge of this disease. (Death as a consequence of measles is generally seen only in undernourished populations.) When doctors started routinely vaccinating children against measles, we started to see babies who contracted measles at a dangerously early age because their vaccinated mothers were not able to pass on immunity to them. And what was the medical community's solution to this dilemma? Vaccinate infants for measles even earlier! Remember that humans are vaccinated only a few times in their lives, whereas animals are so treated once or twice a year for life. Most people with chronically ill animals believe the animals were already sick when they got them, but often we can trace their problems to the time of vaccination (or to their parents having been vaccinated). It's true that vaccinosis does not afflict all vaccinated animals; some are lucky enough to have very strong immune systems. But if you or your animals have ever been affected by it, you'll never forget it. You take a risk every time you allow your animals, your children, or yourself to be vaccinated unnecessarily. Remember, it's your decision, unless the laws in your state complicate your freedom of choice.

Vaccines do not work all the time. In both human and veterinary medicine, there are many recorded instances of no immunity developing, or of so-called "vaccine breaks" occurring, whereby the stimulation of antibodies isn't sufficient to protect against the natural disease. Conventional medicine claims those are body faults and problems. There does appear to be a genetic component to which animals may have trouble responding to a vaccine; a titer test (see "Titers" on page 38) may help distinguish these individuals. However, giving a nonresponding animal more vaccines is unlikely to force an appropriate immune response, and it certainly can cause more problems.

ARE VACCINES NECESSARY?

There has been tremendous overuse of vaccination for many diseases. While still seemingly controversial, it is no longer a theory; virtually every veterinary school and professional organization agrees. The result of the debate, which started in the early 1990s, ultimately produced a poor compromise: boosters every three years instead of annually. However, this is still a bad idea. If a vaccine is effective (and feline panleukopenia, for instance, is known to be an extremely effective vaccine), it produces a large amount of antibodies that circulate in the bloodstream and reside in the lymph nodes for a long time. This is a good thing, because if the cat encounters the natural disease, these antibodies will immediately attack and destroy the virus. However, if a booster vaccine is given while antibodies are present, the same thing happens—the antibodies destroy the virus in the vaccine! It is a basic principle of immunology that booster vaccines do not produce any increase in immunity. In other words, boosters are unnecessary if the original vaccine worked.

CORE VS. NON-CORE VACCINES

Recently veterinary organizations have developed the concept of "core" vaccines that are needed for every animal, and "non-core" vaccines that should only be given under specific circumstances. Core vaccines include feline panleukopenia and rabies (where required by law). All others are non-core and are not recommended for the vast majority of cats. If your veterinarian recommends any non-core vaccines, make sure you understand and agree with her rationale; otherwise, just say no.

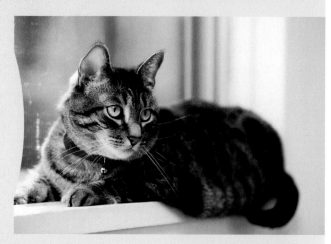

Domestic Shorthair Tabby

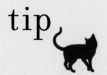

tip

No Scientific Justification for Yearly Boosters!

One-year booster vaccines became the norm by economic consensus among veterinarians and drug companies. As has been pointed out, there is not, and never has been, any scientific justification for yearly boosters. There are many, many studies that demonstrate three-year boosters are just as effective, yet many veterinarians still complain that it hasn't been "proven," and they continue to give every cat every vaccine every year.

VACCINE TIMING

If a mother cat has been vaccinated or has developed immunity due to natural disease, she will secrete antibodies in the first milk (colostrum) suckled by her kittens. These maternal antibodies protect the kittens from dangerous diseases when they are young. These antibodies circulate in the kitten for at least twelve weeks; at that point they gradually break down, while the kitten's own immune system is growing stronger. If the kitten is vaccinated while maternal antibodies are still active, the antibodies will destroy the virus components in the vaccine, and the kitten will not develop its own immunity.

TITERS

A titer measures antibodies in the blood for a specific disease. The blood is diluted, then incubated with a marker of the disease (proteins from a virus, for instance). If antibodies are present, they will react with the marker and produce a positive titer. The most extreme dilution at which the reaction is seen is notated. For example, there may be a reaction to the panleukopenia virus at a dilution factor of 1:1200, which would be a strong positive.

Titers have gained some acceptance as a guideline on whether an animal needs a booster vaccine. For instance, if your cat had a high titer to panleukopenia (or survived it as a kitten), there would be no need to give a booster. There is a growing body of scientific evidence that most viral vaccines produce high, long-lasting titers in most animals.

While titer tests are available for many common diseases, there is no consensus on how high a titer is protective for each disease. While low or borderline titers are open to interpretation, most experts agree that a high titer indicates good protection from the disease. However, titers only measure one part of immunity; a low titer does not always mean the animal does not have immunity to the disease.

If you wish to minimize your cat's vaccines, but want to know—to the extent possible—whether or not she is protected against disease, it may be worthwhile to have your veterinarian run a titer test. It is not perfect, but it does provide a snapshot of at least one important part of the immune system.

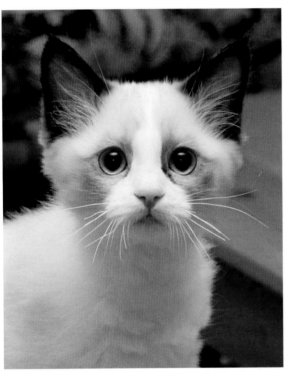

Seal bicolor and white Ragamuffin kitten

Dr. Jean's Perspective on the Rabies Vaccine

Don't skip the rabies vaccine if it's required by law. You need to assess the risks and benefits of the rabies vaccine in your area, as well as consider the legal ramifications of not vaccinating. Wildlife has been known to find its way into homes, creating a small but real risk of exposure even for exclusively indoor cats. The adverse effects of the rabies vaccine are far more common than the disease; on the other hand, the disease will kill you for sure.

Immunologically speaking, a two-vaccine series provides many years or even a lifetime of immunity. Further boosters may be required by law, but they are not necessary for preventing the disease.

It is important for you to know that if your cat bites someone and they go to a doctor, the doctor is legally mandated to report the bite. Animal control will come to your door, and if you cannot show proper proof of current rabies vaccination, your cat can be confiscated and euthanized.

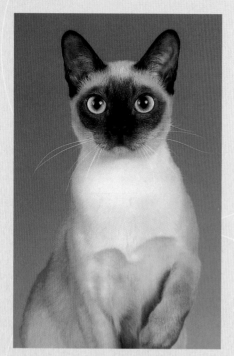

Cat Fanciers' Association's Grand Premier Privatdancer Pansy of Celestecats, Champagne Mink Tonkinese, first generation raw food-fed cat

Celeste's Vaccine Protocol

I have researched this subject quite thoroughly with Dr. Jean and other experts. I also have had a considerable amount of experience in my eleven-generation Tonkinese cat breeding program. Armed with this ammunition, I concluded that there is no absolute solution. What I did —and what all of us must do—is do what works for you.

After considering where I live, the very secure conditions that my indoor cats live in, and the legal issues of where I live (California), I have chosen to give one 3-way, modified live Schering Plough Eclipse 3 vaccine (panleukopenia, rhinotracheitis, and calicivirus) at sixteen weeks of age, and then nothing else further. I have observed that at twelve weeks, the kittens have a very strong response to the vaccine and often become quite ill with severe upper respiratory infections. However, by sixteen weeks, for a day or two they will be "off their food," feel feverish, and then bounce back to their usual rambunctious selves!

I do not have my cats vaccinated for rabies. I am fully aware that there are risks. Dr. Jean's tip box on page 39 discusses rabid wildlife and the danger to cats who could come in contact with them. I take many precautions to prevent the entry of wildlife into my home. I have had great results with my current protocol, coupled with my "ounce of prevention," which keeps my cats exclusively indoors! (Rabies vaccination laws vary from state to state and even town to town. In California, at the time of this writing, the rabies vaccine is recommended, but not required, for cats.)

ARE THERE ALTERNATIVES TO VACCINES?

Some veterinary practitioners advise boosting immunity with nutrition and supplements only. Others prefer homeopathic treatment. In any case, it's certainly true that an undamaged, robust immune system is the best defense against any disease.

VACCINATIONS: THE BOTTOM LINE

If we just continue to accept the practice of vaccination, a safer system will never be developed. Our goal should be to work holistically to keep both ourselves and our cats healthy, period. Here are some tips to consider.

- If you're adopting an older kitten or cat with an unknown vaccine history, you may want to consider a single vaccination for panleukopenia.

- Do not give more than one vaccine at a time; wait at least three weeks between inoculations if you have elected to add another vaccine, such as rabies, to your protocol.

- If you must bring a sick cat to a veterinarian you don't know and that veterinarian wants to vaccinate, it is your right, and duty, to refuse. Every vaccine's instructions state that the vaccine is for use in healthy cats only. These instructions also suggest to not allow other procedures such as surgery or even bathing to be done at the same time, because low body temperatures stress the immune system. Topical flea products should not be applied at the same time; they can cause plenty of their own side effects. (See "Flea Prevention and Treatment" on page 43.) If your cat is to be transported by air, wait at least two weeks to allow recovery from the vaccine and watch for side effects. Make sure your wishes are clearly understood and will be honored.

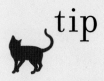

tip

A Matter of Trust

Some veterinarians and vet techs are so convinced of the need for vaccines that they may vaccinate your cat without your permission. If circumstances bring you to a vet you don't trust completely, try not to let the cat out of your sight. Cats have been force-vaccinated when they were taken into the back for a nail-trim, blood draw, or other simple procedure. In many cases, the first time the people notice it is on the invoice for payment, and then it's too late. It is also a good idea to state that you are not interested in topical flea products, because they may automatically use a topical on your cat. Be sure your wishes are clearly stated in your file as well as saying it directly to your veterinarian. You are your cat's first and last line of defense, so stay alert!

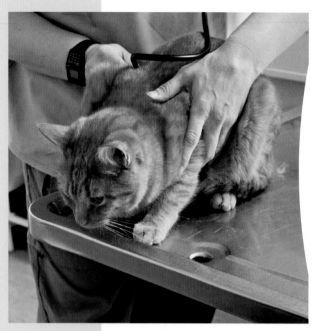

Domestic Shorthair Tabby getting a routine checkup

A CLOSE LOOK AT CONVENTIONAL VETERINARY MEDICAL TREATMENT

Medical science, whether conventional or alternative, human or veterinary, is constantly changing as new information becomes available. As with vaccines, new research can shed light on drugs and treatments that have long been used without that full understanding.

ANTIBIOTICS

The overuse and misuse of antibiotics is widespread. An estimated 70 percent of antibiotics in the United States are administered to livestock who are destined for the human and pet food supply. Veterinarians contribute to this cycle when they prescribe antibiotics for viral infections, cystitis (bladder inflammation), and other diseases where they are clearly not necessary. (Antibiotics are only effective against bacteria, not against viruses.)

If your cat genuinely needs antibiotics, it's crucial to simultaneously supplement with probiotics ("friendly" gut bacteria). *Antibiotic* means "against life," and these drugs don't discriminate—they kill the good bacteria as well as the bad and the ugly! To prevent diarrhea and other tummy problems, repopulating the good bacteria helps minimize side effects of the drugs. Continue probiotics for at least thirty days after the antibiotics are stopped. (See "Supplements and Whole Food Products" in Resources on page 174 for suppliers.)

STEROIDS

Steroids suppress the immune system. They do not cure disease; they just mask the symptoms. Repeated doses are needed to maintain the effect. There are cases in which steroid use is justified. A short course of oral steroids (five to seven days) or a short-acting injection can be effective as a diagnostic tool as well as for pain management. However, think long and hard before you agree to condemn your cat to a lifetime of steroids for asthma, food allergies, arthritis, or inflammatory bowel disease. There are many alternative treatments for these conditions, so consult your holistic vet if steroids have been recommended for your cat.

The steroids most frequently used in veterinary medicine are powerful anti-inflammatories; they include cortisone, prednisone, prednisolone, dexamethosone, and triamcinolone. There are two things you should know about steroids:

- Cats should only be given prednisolone in oral form, never prednisone, because it's less stressful to the liver.

- Injectable "depot" steroids (such as depomedrol), where the effect lasts for weeks, can cause diabetes, even from the very first injection. (The oral forms are less likely to do this.)

Other side effects of steroids include increased appetite, weight gain, increased thirst, increased urination, high blood pressure, impaired wound healing, muscle weakness, thinning of skin, immune suppression (increased risk of infection), stomach ulcers, heart disease, hypertension, and psychological/behavior changes.

PAIN MEDICATIONS

A cat's liver has very limited capacity to process drugs, which makes it difficult to design a pharmaceutical pain management protocol for more than about three days, which is the longest safe interval for most drugs. Here is an area where alternative medicine really shines—homeopathy and herbs (see chapter 5), acupuncture and energy work (see chapter 6), nutraceuticals (see chapter 7). Specific nutritional supplementation, such as glucosamine and MSM (for arthritis), and many other modalities are excellent pain reducers that increase mobility and simply make life more comfortable. Contact your holistic vet to tailor a program for your cat.

FLEA PREVENTION AND TREATMENT

Flea collars (whether herbal or insecticidal) don't work! They don't kill fleas, and they don't even particularly repel them, except for the area right around the collar. The grocery/pet store variety contains concentrated toxic chemicals, and the herbal ones are irritating to odor-sensitive cats. Topical (spot-on or pour-on) flea preventatives are associated with liver disease and other adverse effects in cats. Permethrin, pyrethrin, or pyrethroid-containing products intended for dogs are extremely toxic to cats and have caused many feline

deaths. Putting a dog product on a cat causes neurological signs (twitching, disorientation, seizures) that ultimately kill about 10 percent of cats.

Healthy cats eating a balanced raw diet are much less susceptible to fleas and other parasites. If your cat is experiencing a flea problem, work on improving your cat's overall health and deal with the immediate parasite situation. This is a "holistic" approach in the truest sense of the word! The conventional thinking that fleas are the problem is like saying "flies cause garbage" just because the two are often found together. It is the unhealthy state of the animal that attracts the parasites, just like garbage attracts flies.

Fleas, those nasty little blood suckers, are tough, highly evolved parasites that, once entrenched, are not easily eliminated. Fleas are attracted to warmth, moving shadows, and the vibrations from foot (or paw) steps. When dealing with fleas, you need to protect your cat and reach fleas and larvae hiding in carpets and yards. Even exclusively indoor cats can get fleas, which travel in on shoes and clothing. (Keeping your cat indoors, however, will eliminate the risk of ticks.) And removing shoes at your front door keeps fleas out and helps keep other germs out as well.

Adult fleas spend most of their time on the cat, where they feed on blood several times a day. Flea eggs are slippery and quickly fall off the cat and onto the cat's resting areas, floors, rugs, bedding, and furniture. The eggs hatch and go through several intermediate stages before emerging as adults in as little as two weeks, but they may remain dormant for months. That's why even if you get rid of the fleas on your cat, reinfestation is a common and very frustrating phenomenon.

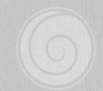

A Three-Pronged Approach to Treating Fleas

Try this one-two-three punch to eradicate fleas from your—and your cat's—life.

ON YOUR CAT:

🌀 Use an ultra-fine-tooth flea comb daily. Pay particular attention to the neck, tummy, and base of the tail, which are favorite flea hangouts. Have a glass or bowl full of warm, soapy water at hand to drown any fleas that turn up.

🌀 Bathe your cat. Bathing your cat will drown a lot of fleas, but apply soap around the ears and neck first to keep the fleas from rushing up to the cat's head and face. The herb *Erigeron Canadensis* (Canadian fleabane), found in some herbal shampoos, will help kill fleas. Bathe no more than once a week. (See "Cleaning and Pest Control" in Resources on page 174 for some suppliers.)

IN YOUR HOME:

🌀 Floor/carpet treatments such as diatomaceous earth (the fossilized shells of one-celled organisms called diatoms) and boric acid–derived powders will kill flea larvae, primarily through dessication (drying). Exterminators use borates; you can either hire professionals to treat your home or do it yourself. For a serious flea problem, it may be worth paying a professional since their work is guaranteed. (See "Cleaning and Pest Control" in Resources on page 174 for some suppliers.)

🌀 Vacuuming is very effective against flea eggs and might even catch a few adults. To keep the eggs from hatching or the fleas from escaping, discard the bag immediately or use a flea spray in the vacuum bag or container, either before or right after you vacuum.

IN THE YARD:

🌀 Beneficial nematodes eat flea eggs and will help control flea populations outdoors.

🌀 Garden-grade diatomaceous earth is very effective. Concentrate on areas under shrubs and decks and other cool shady spots where animals (such as rodents, raccoons, and outdoor and feral cats) have access.

TOXINS IN YOUR HOME

There are many reasons to create a nontoxic environment in your home—obviously, the health of self, family, and companion animals are at the top of the list. Over time, exposure to toxic chemicals can contribute to the development of cancer, birth defects, genetic changes, allergies, and other disorders and illnesses, to say nothing of a generally weakened immune system.

Children and pets are the most vulnerable to toxicity, owing to their size and physiology. Their smaller size translates to a higher rate of metabolism, including heart and breathing rates. Many pollutants are heavier than air and are therefore found in greater concentration lower to the ground, so children and animals receive much higher exposure.

CLEANING PRODUCTS

Ironically, cleaning products are among the most hazardous materials found in the home. Many household items on the market are mislabeled or lack adequate warnings. Consider replacing the following with nontoxic, biodegradable substitutes.

- Air fresheners
- Detergents
- Disinfectant
- Fabric softener
- Furniture polish
- Glass cleaner
- Insecticides
- Scouring powder

CAT-SAFE INGREDIENTS

Check your local health food store for safe products, or make your own from the following cat-safe ingredients.

INGREDIENT	PURPOSE
Aromatherapy hydrosols	Air fresheners
Baking soda	Deodorizer and nonscratch scouring cleanser; use as a paste with water for polishing metals
Beeswax	Polish for floors and furniture
Bleach	**(diluted 1:32 or 1 ounce in 1 gallon of water (30 mls per 4L)** Still the best disinfectant; kills bacteria and viruses; once dry is totally safe.
Borax	Deodorizer; nonscratch scouring cleanser; mold inhibitor; flea-egg killer; removes rust stains
Jojoba oil	Furniture polish
Lavender oil	Disinfectant, antibacterial
Lemon juice	Grease-cutting cleanser, deodorizer
Neem tree oil	Antibacterial, insect repellent
Vinegar, white distilled	Grease-cutting cleanser for floors and hard surfaces; glass cleaner; deodorizes and disinfects; natural fabric softener; kills fungus and mold
Toothpaste (not gel)	Silver and other metal polish

PBDEs and Hyperthyroidism

A recent study suggests that fire-retardant chemicals known as Polybrominated diphenyl ethers (PBDEs) may be a factor in feline hyperthyroidism. PBDEs were introduced to consumer goods at about the same time hyperthyroidism was first described in cats. Additionally, the rate of feline hyperthyroidism has roughly paralleled the use of PBDEs worldwide. The main route of exposure in cats is hypothesized to be the PBDEs contained in carpets, upholstery, and mattresses—and the dust mites that live in these fabrics. Electronic equipment, which attracts dust, is also a suspect. Since cats often sleep on carpets, sofas, chairs, mattresses, and warm TVs, computer monitors, and stereos, their exposure could be high and prolonged. Subsequent grooming would then cause the cat to ingest a fairly large amount of dust. This may explain why hyperthyroidism is also more common in indoor cats.

SMOKE

Smoke from cigarettes, cigars, pipes, and other smoking materials is highly toxic to your cat. All smoking must be done outside and well away from doors and windows to minimize smoke drifting back into the house. Smoke contains toxic chemicals that will settle onto furniture, floors, and other objects. Even with these precautions, toxic dust clings to skin and clothing, and it can be transferred to your cat by petting or by contact with contaminated fabric. Ultimately, it will be ingested by the cat.

COMMERCIAL PET FOODS

The global commercial pet food industry is astonishingly profitable and continues to grow (sadly) by leaps and bounds. Hundreds of generations of pet guardians have fed their animals successfully without processed pet food, but that fact has been virtually forgotten by consumers.

Conventional thinking causes us to pose the question, "How can we trust the feeding of our beloved companions to an industry driven by profit?" Keeping prices competitive requires the use of cheap ingredients. To make these inferior ingredients appeal to pets, artificial colors and flavors are added. The consumer saves money on pet food in the short run, but ultimately will incur enormous veterinary bills to treat problems that could have been prevented with better nutrition.

Many commercial pet food companies label their products misleadingly. Processed wood chips are called "powdered cellulose," and a ground-up array of disease-ridden tissue and unwanted animal parts—often containing high levels of hormones, antibiotics, and pesticides—are labeled as "meat and bone meal."

The percentages of protein, fat, and carbohydrates listed on the labels provide little or no useful information on whether or not the ingredients are bioavailable—that is, can our pets digest *and* use them in their bodies?

If our cats keeled over and died after they ate a bowl of kibble or a single can of commercial food—as unfortunately many did in the massive worldwide 2007 pet food recall, and there have been dozens of recalls before and since then—there would be no doubt about its danger. However, since it takes years to develop cancer and other degenerative diseases, most allopathic veterinarians never make the connection between diet and chronic disease. Put bluntly, commercial pet foods may sustain life, but they don't promote health.

Here are some basic facts about commercial pet food ingredients and labeling.

BY-PRODUCTS

Even on "premium" and "super-premium" brand labels, one of the major ingredients listed is by-products of some sort. By-products are used primarily in canned pet foods. By-products are basically "parts other than meat." These may include internal organs not commonly eaten by humans, such as lungs, spleens, and intestines; other parts such as cow udders and uteri; and in the case of poultry by-products, undeveloped eggs, beaks, and feet. While it's true that a cat would eat by-products in its natural diet when it consumes an entire bird or mouse, these entrails should not be relied on to the exclusion of meat.

RENDERED PRODUCTS

Rendering (basically a slow-cooking process) produces two significant ingredients: animal fat or tallow and a processed "meal" product. The latter may be called meat meal, meat-and-bone meal, or by-product meal depending on its composition. Due to historical quirks in naming, the term by-product meal refers to poultry, while the equivalent mammalian product is called "meat and bone meal." Rendered products are found primarily in dry pet foods.

Animals that are dead, dying, diseased, or disabled prior to reaching the slaughterhouse are known as "downers" or "4D" animals. These are usually condemned, in whole or in part, for human consumption, and they are generally sent for rendering along with other by-products, parts and items that are unwanted or unsuitable for human use—such as out-of-date supermarket meats (including their plastic wrappers), cut-away cancerous tissue, and fetal tissue (which is very high in hormones).

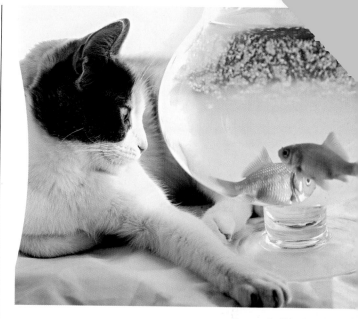

Domestic Shorthair

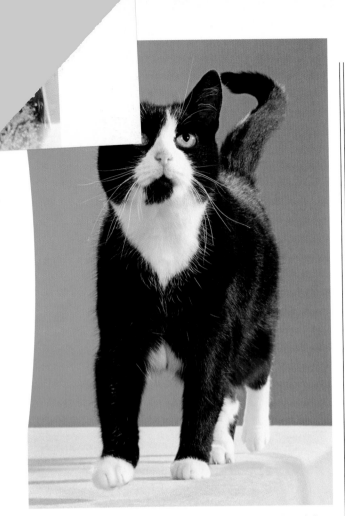

Black and White Domestic Shorthair "Tuxedo" cat

"COMPLETE AND BALANCED" CLAIMS

A food may be labeled as "complete and balanced" if it meets the standards set by the Association of American Feed Control Officials. These standards were formulated in the early 1990s by panels of canine and feline nutrition experts. State Feed Control Officials (or equivalent authorities) are then responsible for enforcement, though, in many cases, enforcement is negligible. The standards set only minimums and maximums, not optimums. The danger of conventional thinking is that minimums are good enough for our pets' health.

ADDITIVES AND PRESERVATIVES

Virtually every commercial pet food contains additives and preservatives. Dry foods and soft-moist foods contain additives to produce the colors, shapes, and textures of the food. Canned foods typically contain coloring and flavoring agents. Some of the worst preservatives, found primarily in dry foods, include Butylated hydroxyanisole (BHA), butylated hydroxytoluene (BHT), propyl gallate, and ethoxyquin. Ethoxyquin is banned from nearly all human food products (except certain spices) due to its cancer-causing properties. *Warning:* Be sure to read labels on everything that goes into your companion animal's mouth. For instance, the preservative sodium benzoate, which is added to some food products as well as many brands of aloe vera juice, is known to be exceptionally poisonous to cats. Look for brands free of this dangerous preservative. (See "Supplements and Whole Food Products" in Resources on page 174 for some suppliers.)

Rendered ingredients vary greatly in quality. A few rendering facilities are closely associated with slaughterhouses, which are in turn connected with feedlots or poultry farms. These "captive" rendering plants, which do not accept outside materials, are more likely to produce decent quality, single-species meat meals. Such meals are typically designated with the name of the source animal, such as "chicken meal."

Many consumers are now aware of what "meat and bone meal" indicates on a pet food label. As a result, some manufacturers are now calling this ingredient "beef and bone meal" and similarly euphemistic terms.

Fact or Fiction: Pets *in* Pet Food?

Over the years, there have been numerous unsubstantiated reports of euthanized cats and dogs being processed into pet food. The Center for Veterinary Medicine, a branch of the U.S. Food and Drug Administration (FDA), admits that dead dogs and cats are commonly rendered, and although there is no legal prohibition against using dogs and cats in pet food, they do not condone the practice.

This allegation was undoubtedly true at some point, but today all reputable pet food manufacturers certify that they do not allow such materials in their products. Whether or not the renderers who supply the pet food companies are complying is unknown. Renderers would be extremely foolish to jeopardize profitable pet food contracts when these materials can be put to many other uses.

Animal remains can be turned into fertilizer, industrial lubricants, cosmetics, soaps, tires, asphalt, glue, film, or any of hundreds of other products. (However, as fertilizer, this material can be introduced into the human food supply, the by-products of which become pet food.)

The FDA conducted a study to determine whether or not the "pets in pet food" story was true. They searched for the euthanasia drug sodium pentobarbital in dry dog foods—the most likely foods to contain it. They found plenty of it, primarily in foods containing meat and bone meal, animal fat, beef and bone meal, and animal digest. However, the FDA attributed the presence of the drug to euthanized livestock. The FDA claims that the amounts are too low to cause a problem; however, the long-term health implications of consuming this drug are completely unknown. The FDA further used a test it developed to check for dog and cat DNA in the foods, and found none. So although it is certain that many pet foods used to contain these cannibalistic materials, the industry does appear to have cleaned up its act. Does that mean that we can trust that never happens? No, and the pet food makers cannot guarantee it since they are relying on the trustworthiness of the notoriously secretive rendering industry.

Ultimately, we all should ask ourselves, "Why trust big business to make our pets' food when it is so easy to do it ourselves and insure the ingredients used meet our own standards?" (See chapter 4.)

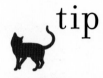

tip

Take Control of Your Pet's Remains

To insure that your humanely euthanized pet may rest in peace where you deem appropriate and does not become processed at a rendering plant, you must make arrangements with your vet to take control of your pet's remains. Your vet may recommend a reliable cremation or pet burial facility if local laws prohibit pet burial on your own property.

It is also important to know that if your vet sends your animals' remains to a facility to be necropsied, you can pay a little extra to have your pet's remains cremated after necropsy, and the ashes sent back to you. Otherwise, the remains may be picked up by disposal trucks and taken to rendering plants. (See "Pet Loss" in Resources on page 174 for a pet cremation facility to which people can ship frozen remains overnight.)

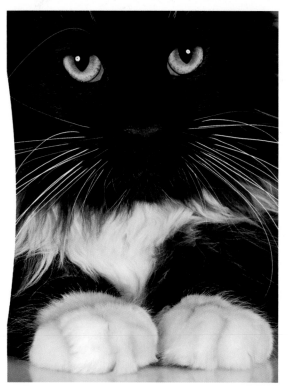

Black and White Domestic Longhair

CONTAMINANTS

Pesticide residues, antibiotics, and molds are often found in pet food ingredients. Meat from downer animals may be loaded with drugs, some of which are known to pass unchanged through all the processing done to create a finished pet food. Grain products condemned for human consumption due to excessive pesticide residue can be used without limit in food intended for animals.

There are also deliberate contaminants, such as melamine in wheat gluten and rice protein from China that was implicated in the deaths of tens of thousands of pets in 2007. The use of melamine to falsely elevate the protein levels in many food products is a widespread practice in China despite its illegality. Since 2007, melamine has been found in dozens of Chinese-made human food products around the world such as infant formula and milk chocolate.

As decent quality ingredients become scarcer and far more expensive, look for more problems from imported foods—including big-name brands manufactured far from the company's home office. The bottom line? Dry pet foods are the likeliest to contain unwanted ingredients and contaminants that have no place in the feline diet. If you take only one piece of advice in this entire book, please let it be to stop feeding dry food.

MODERN CONVENIENCES AND YOUR CAT'S HEALTH

Millions of dollars are spent convincing us we can't live without this or that modern convenience, without regard for the consequences to our health, or to that of our cats.

MICROWAVE OVENS

The microwave is high on the list of lethal "conveniences." A Swiss study indicated that human consumption of microwaved milk and vegetables was associated with a rise in cholesterol and a decline in hemoglobin levels. Low levels of hemoglobin are associated with anemia, which may result in rheumatism, fever, and thyroid insufficiency. The study also concluded that eating microwaved vegetables was associated with a major drop in lymphocyte (a type of white blood cell) counts, showing that the subjects tested were responding to the food as if it were an infectious agent. The subjects' radiation levels of light-emitting bacteria were higher as well, which indicated that microwave energy was being transmitted from food to person. This is to say nothing of the damage done to food when it is violently vibrated at 2.5 million times per second. Conclusion: Never warm cat food in the microwave.

Why Most Fish Is Bad for Cats

A lot of cats love fish, and conventional thinking says it's great, but it's really not a good idea to feed fish to your cat! Here's why.

- The fish used in canned pet foods usually includes bones and are high in phosphorus and magnesium, which can be an issue in cats with a history of urinary tract disorders or kidney disease. Quite a few cats develop urinary tract infections and blockages if they eat fish—even boneless fish.

- Many cats are sensitive or even allergic to fish; it is one of the most common food allergens.

- Fish tends to be "addictive" to cats. They love it and will often stage a hunger strike by refusing their regular food in favor of fish.

- There is a known link between the feeding of fish-based canned cat foods and the development of hyperthyroidism in older cats.

- Predatory fish at the top of the food chain, such as tuna and salmon, may contain very elevated levels of heavy metals (including mercury) as well as PCBs, pesticides, and other toxins. Tilefish (listed on pet food labels as "ocean whitefish") are among the worst contaminated, along with king mackerel, shark, and swordfish. These fish are so toxic that the FDA advises that women of child-bearing age and children should avoid them entirely, and the FDA recommends only one serving of albacore tuna per week due to its high mercury levels.

- The vast majority of salmon today comes from factory-farmed fish. These unfortunate animals are kept in overcrowded pens in polluted coastal waters. They're fed antifungals, antibiotics, and brightly colored dyes to make their flesh salmon colored; it is naturally gray. Common water pollutants such as PCBs, pesticides, and other chemicals are present in farmed salmon at ten times the amount found in wild fish. These contaminants will be present in any product made with farmed fish, including cat and dog food.

In general, a small amount of fish, such as sardines or herring, used as a flavoring, or as a source of omega 3 fatty acid, is not a problem, but fish should not be a mainstay of any cat's diet.

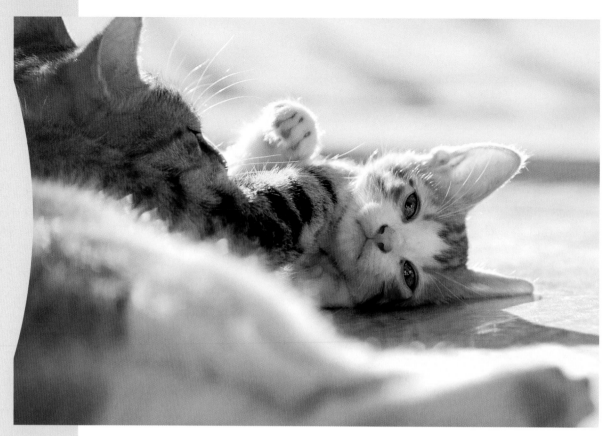

Domestic Shorthair Tabbies

TAP WATER

Fluoride, which is added to tap water in many municipalities, is thought by many experts to be more poisonous than lead and just slightly less poisonous than arsenic. It accumulates in bone over the years, and can, in sensitive individuals, cause skin eruptions such as atopic dermatitis, as well as gastric distress and weakness in some people. Be sure to tell your veterinary dentist that you do not want your cat treated with fluoride. (See "The Importance of Pure Drinking Water" on page 78 for more information on safe water for your cats.)

ELECTROMAGNETIC FIELDS

All plants and animals operate by tiny electrochemical pulses at about the same frequency as the energy field on the planet. We are all virtually swimming daily in a pool of electromagnetic chaos. Our cell phones, telephone lines, computers, battery chargers, televisions, and so on all produce toxic electromagnetic fields (EMFs). Excessive EMFs are thought to cause cancer, birth defects, cataracts, heart disease, and other health problems.

Be aware of the lights you use in your home. As energy-efficient as our new bulbs may be, or as attractive as incandescent lighting is in our homes, there is nothing more beneficial than natural light. Full spectrum light provides relief from Seasonal Affective Disorder (SAD) in people.

ANTIFREEZE AND OTHER TOXINS

A tiny amount (¼ teaspoon [about 1 ml]) of antifreeze (ethylene glycol) has a lethal effect on cats, triggering slow and painful kidney failure. Symptoms of antifreeze poisoning include agitation and vomiting, followed days later by general decline, coma, and death. Even an indoor cat is at risk if she has access to a garage and there has been a leak under a car. If antifreeze comes into contact with her paws, she will lick it off (due to the meticulous nature of cats). Keep all toxic chemicals safely secured in your garage, including rat poisons, snail pellets, and garden fertilizers. Better yet, explore environmentally safe alternatives to these toxic substances.

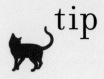

tip

Depleted Negative Ions

The artificial world we have created for ourselves and our pets deprives us of the sensory pleasure of negative ions. Negative ions, which have beneficial effects on the immune and nervous systems, are experienced during rain, at the sea shore, near a waterfall or in a forest; positive ions are found more in desert habitats and where there is a lot of concrete. Himalayan salt lamps are one means of releasing negative ions naturally into our environment.

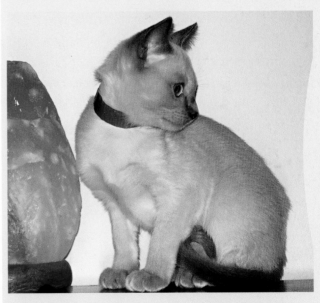

Celestecats Tonkinese kitten with a Himalayan salt lamp

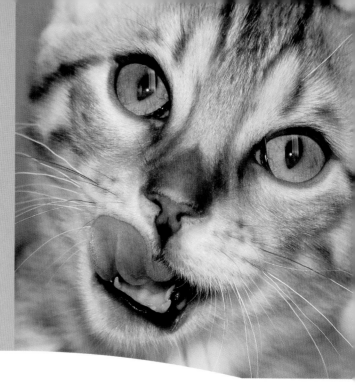

CHAPTER

4

NUTRITION AS PREVENTATIVE MEDICINE

Domestic Shorthair Tabby

Eating right is the key to good health and longevity for people, and it's the same for cats. Vitality, contentment, and zest for life come from within. They spring from a body and brain that are fully supplied with essential nutrients in the right form. The best nutrition provides the cat's body what it needs, not just to survive but to thrive, without burdening the body with indigestible waste, chemical additives, or other harmful substances. To live out her longest life in the best health, your cat needs to eat well. In this chapter, we'll show you exactly how to help her do that.

Cats are hardwired to hunt. We see them perched in their window seats chattering at the birds (they're actually practicing their killing bites with this funny little action), but few cat companions actually know that cats have fixed neural circuits in their brains that make the stalking action and grabbing their prey a reflex behavior. All it takes is for an object to move, and the hunting switch flips on—just like a light switch. This is a profound experience for the cat—any size cat. Cats have incredible hearing that allows them to hear the ultrasonic calls of rodents and insects. When the cat is hunting, the auditory nerves are extremely active. But once the cat locks onto the prey visually and prepares to pounce, auditory nerve activity stops. In that moment, the feline goes deaf. The cat's body enters sensory shutdown mode, which enables its whole being to focus on the prey.

THE CAT'S NATURAL DIET

The feline has emerged through the stages of evolution as an obligate carnivore, which means that all cats—from the tiny pedigreed Singapura cat to the Bengal tiger—are creatures whose carnivorous nature is 100 percent dependant on their species-specific diet: fresh raw prey. Cats also relish certain insects (like crickets), which are tiny, high protein snacks to round out their meal plans.

Everything about the cat, from its unique physiology to its behavior, demonstrates that what it needs to achieve optimum health depends on fulfilling its strict dietary requirements.

THE CARNIVORE'S TEETH

A cat's mouth contains four long teeth called canines at the front of the jaws. He has sharp serrated teeth at the back of the jaw, which are used to grasp and tear the meat from the bones. These teeth contain an array of pressure-sensitive nerves. When a cat grips a mouse with his canines, his teeth find the space between the mouse's vertebrae and deliver a quick, clean, killing bite. Remember, in the wild, the cat only gets to eat and feed its young when they win the battle and manage not to have dinner whisked away by another predator. Survival of the fittest is the law of the jungle even if the jungle is your own kitchen.

The cat has adapted physiologically to getting many of its nutritional needs met secondhand through the prey animal's digestive processes. On the other hand, the cat has myriad other receptors for certain chemicals found in their meal of raw meat. Cats can taste if their meat is fresh killed, or if it comes from the meat department of your local health food store. Cats know (in their brainstem and cerebellum, which govern instinctual survival behaviors and thinking) whether the prey is a minute or a day from its end. They may even be able to detect how the prey died if they didn't kill it themselves.

Cats, if given the choice, would prefer their mice to our modern packaged meat. We are not suggesting that you turn your housecats out into the wild and allow them to fend for themselves. A mouse in your domain may seem like a golden opportunity to test your cat's natural instincts. Please use caution! Many house mice have ingested rat poison, and field mice can carry infectious diseases and parasites.

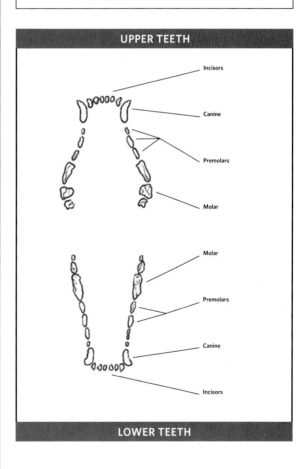

THE CARNIVORE'S TEETH

UPPER TEETH

Incisors

Canine

Premolars

Molar

Molar

Premolars

Canine

Incisors

LOWER TEETH

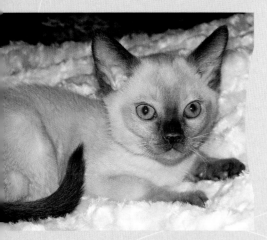

Butch, a Celestecats Champagne Mink Tonkinese, ninth generation raw food–fed kitten

Butch's Instincts

Butch was precocious, even as a kitten. He was the first in his ninth generation litter of naturally-raised Celestecats Tonkinese kittens to sample his mom's raw meat meal at the age of five weeks. He was the first to abscond with a piece of raw chicken neck, shred, tear, and crunch it just like his mom would do. Kittens raised on a properly prepared raw meat diet generally have phenomenal appetites, but Butch was something else. He had a great little spirit and sense of play that made everyone who met him fall in love at first sight.

When Butch was sixteen weeks old, his human parents adopted him. After a brief period of adjustment, Butch quickly ruled their roost. These folks loved animals—all kinds of animals—and even kept a pet snake. "Snakey" had his own room and habitat where he was occasionally fed live mice. Butch discovered how to sneak in to this room, unbeknownst to the humans, to watch this feeding ritual. One fine day, the mouse got away. Butch sprang into action. Every muscle coiled, and quivering slightly, with a flick of his tail—Wham! Pounce! He got him! It was an incredible sight for the snake and the human!

Almost all cats can catch mice, or any other small creature for that matter. According to all the cat experts, Butch was not supposed to know how to dissect the prey, let alone eat it once he caught it. Allegedly a mother cat, who was taught by her mother, must teach her kittens to hunt and then eat their dinner. Butch's mother is a beautiful Tonkinese lap cat, retired from the show ring and breeding program, who never saw a mouse in her entire life. Butch toyed with the mouse for a few minutes, flipping him up in the air (this is not really play; it is a tenderization procedure facilitating dissection), and finally ending with a little snack for himself. Now, Butch waits at the door every day, often bringing the rest of his cat friends to watch. It finally became evident to his human parents that perhaps Butch needed to have his own mouse adventure from time to time. He has tried to give mouse catching lessons to the other cats, but they seem to prefer the snake's cricket treats. Butch remains the only mouse catcher in the family.

DRY FOOD: ONE CONVENIENCE YOU NEED TO DO WITHOUT

When cats first began to live with humans and rely on us for their food, they took a huge and risky step. This is because the feline is completely dependent on his prey for his nutrients. The feline has discarded many important biochemical mechanisms that would allow adaptation to other foods (such as carbohydrates, which in nature would only be found in their predigested form in the prey animal's gut). The feline is bound by his obligate carnivore nature, and he thrives only on meat-based foods. Why then do we see so many carbohydrates in commercial pet food? Unfortunately, real meat is very expensive, and commercial pet food makers must limit their costs to make a profit.

Dental disease is also a common health problem seen by veterinarians; nearly every cat will have it to some degree by the age of three. Of course, nearly every cat is eating commercial pet food. Dry food manufacturers claim their kibble (or treat) keeps cats' teeth clean. But cats mainly shred, tear, and bone-crunch their food. Some cats will gnaw on dry food, but for the most part they swallow dry food whole. In fact, the kibbles are deliberately made small enough to do just that. There's little scientific evidence to support any benefit of dry food to the cat or its teeth.

CATS AND HYDRATION

Cats evolved on the dry African savannahs, and they have a low thirst drive. They don't voluntarily drink water until they are significantly dehydrated. In the wild, cats get most of their water from their food. Cats drink by rapidly dipping their tongues into the water and drawing it back into their mouths; it is not an efficient way to consume water. Animals such as horses and other ruminants suck water up into their mouths; they must be efficient drinkers because they eat a diet primarily consisting of dry forage.

Nutrition-Related Conditions

Dry food may be convenient, but there's a terrible trade-off: your cat's health and well-being. If good nutrition is compromised, your cat is likely to develop one of the following dry-food-related syndromes:

- Obesity
- Diabetes
- Chronic vomiting
- Constipation
- Chronic diarrhea
- Hepatic lipidosis (liver failure)
- Pancreatitis
- Arthritis
- Heart disease
- Asthma
- Allergies
- Inflammatory bowel disease
- Chronic renal failure
- Lower urinary tract disease
- Hyperthyroidism
- High blood pressure
- Viral conjunctivitis
- Skin and coat problems
- Cancer

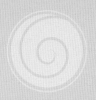

Feline Obesity

At least 25 percent of cats in the United States and Europe are overweight; some statistics suggest that the number is quickly rising and may actually be more than 50 percent. Weight is a contributing factor to nearly all of the diet-related diseases listed on page 57. Fat cells produce inflammation, and chronic inflammation ultimately produces disease.

Free-choice feeding of dry food is the single biggest factor affecting our cats' weight. Getting cats off of dry food and onto a more appropriate diet is the key to weight control. (See "The Paw System" on pages 67.)

The following Body Condition Chart will help you assess—and face the reality of—your cat's weight. It's important to have an idea of your cat's starting point. The homemade diet recipe in this chapter will help your cat achieve his perfect weight; you can use this chart to assess his progress.

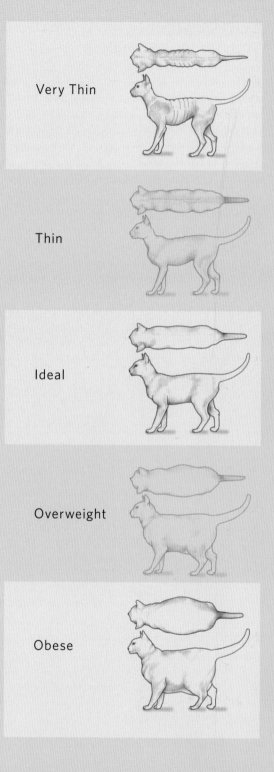

Very Thin

Thin

Ideal

Overweight

Obese

The feline's urine is extremely concentrated. Its natural diet—prey animals—contains 65 to 70 percent water. That means that for every one part of solids or "dry matter," the cat is taking in two parts of water. Cats eating dry kibble (90 percent dry matter and only 10 percent moisture) need to drink twice as much water as the food they are eating to obtain the same ratio of water to dry matter. The problem is that they don't. In fact, cats eating dry food—even though they're the ones you see drinking water—actually take in only half the amount of moisture as a cat eating a wet diet similar in water content to its natural prey.

FELINE LOWER URINARY TRACT DISEASE

Feline Lower Urinary Tract Disease (FLUTD) is a term used to describe a variety of bladder conditions in cats, including idiopathic cystitis (similar to human bladder infections), crystals, stones, and blockages. FLUTD affects less than 3 percent of cats, but it is one of the most common ailments for which cats see a veterinarian.

FLUTD occurs mainly in cats fed a diet of either partially or completely of dry food (kibble). It is more common in overweight cats. Cystitis is annoying and painful for cats, as they constantly try to pass a few drops of urine. Urinary blockages can be fatal in male cats, since toxic waste builds up in the blood instead of being filtered out through the urine.

In FLUTD, inflammation continually stimulates the nerves in the bladder wall, making the cat feel as though its bladder were full, which results in frequent attempts to urinate. Stones, crystals, blood, and mucus secreted by the bladder lining can cause a plug in a male cat's long, narrow urethra, blocking the outflow of urine from the bladder. A urinary blockage is life-threatening and requires emergency care.

SYMPTOMS OF FLUTD INCLUDE THE FOLLOWING:

- Straining to urinate
- Frequent and/or prolonged attempts to urinate
- Crying out while urinating
- Excessive licking of the genital area
- Urinating outside the litter box
- Blood in the urine

If you observe any of these symptoms, get your cat to the vet immediately. This is painful and distressing to your cat, and it can be a very serious and potentially life-threatening situation (especially for males).

If your cat suffers from FLUTD, let your vet know that you'd like to put your cat on the species-appropriate diet. You may be offered a dry prescription diet that contains an acidifier. This may help short term, but about half of cats remaining on dry food will have one or more relapses within a year. Canned food is a better choice, and holistic vets have seen even more spectacular results on a raw food diet.

The natural diet for the cat is wet food, which should consist of raw meat or poultry along with appropriate supplements such as calcium and other vitamins and minerals. (See "Basic Fresh Raw Food Recipe" on page 70.) Nature provides the obligate carnivore with meat, and meat produces a low (acidic) urinary pH (about 6.5). This, along with the higher percentage of water in the food, keeps urine flowing through the system, and it helps prevent crystals and stones of all types from forming.

Melamine and Wheat Gluten

The melamine-laced wheat gluten that caused the 2007 pet food recalls of canned and dry food puzzled most consumers. Why was a known allergen that is not an essential nutrient added to so many brands of cat food? The purpose of gluten is to thicken "gravy" and provide structure and stability to slices, nuggets, chunks, and other molded bits. It's also known as "textured vegetable protein."

Carbohydrates are much cheaper than protein and even fat, which increases profits for the commercial food companies. When all the various nonmeat items on commercial labels are added up, they often outweigh the meat ration. Despite label claims, meat is not the main source of protein in dry food. The food is good for the stockholders, but not so good for your cat!

CATS AND CARBOHYDRATES DO NOT MIX

In most mammals, carbohydrate digestion begins in the mouth with the enzyme amylase that is secreted in saliva; you have to chew for a while to distribute the enzyme. Not only do cats lack salivary amylase, they don't chew! Cats, after they shred, tear, and bone crush, for the most part swallow their food in large chunks. Cats have no dietary need for carbohydrates (except as young kittens, which is why there is lactose in feline milk). Most other mammals (humans included) use carbohydrates as their bodies' "highest octane" fuel. For these animals, the energy system is based on an enzyme called glucokinase, which we think of as the feast or famine mechanism. This system is used by athletes who "carbo-load" (eat a big pasta dinner the night before an event). The glucokinase system is kicked into high gear, sending a massive dose of energy to the body, which in the athlete's case is stored in the liver and muscles as glycogen. The day of the race, the body has extra glycogen to use as fuel—a big advantage for the athlete.

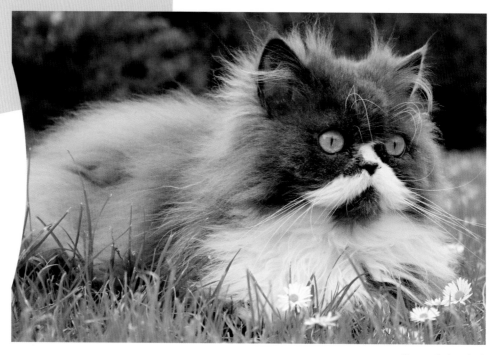

Domestic Longhair

Cats do not operate on the glucokinase enzyme system; they use protein and fat directly for energy. The small amount of carbohydrate they get in their natural diet is handled by hexokinase, an enzyme system that cannot speed up to handle large meals or slow down during a fasting interval. When fed carbs such as those found in most dry foods, cats store them primarily as fat, not glycogen. The purpose of carbohydrates in commercial cat foods is a source of "energy," which simply means calories. For cats, these carbs are mostly empty calories. (This is why cats that eat dry food so often get fat!)

The cat uses dietary fat and protein for energy; if these are not supplied, it must break down fat and protein stored within its own body. Be it wild or tame, large or small, the cat's basic structure and function have not changed through the ages.

ESSENTIAL NUTRIENTS FOR CATS

When preparing a homemade raw food diet (as you will learn to do in the following pages), it's vital to remember that cats cannot live on meat alone. There are many case histories of unfortunate cats who suffered and died from being fed only meat (or fish or liver). As an example, there is virtually no calcium in meat. A cat fed a meat-only diet must satisfy its calcium requirement by stealing from its own bones and ultimately can fracture a leg just walking across a room.

Using the prey animal as our model, and taking into account the vitamins and minerals found not only in its meat but its blood, bones, glands, and organs, we can formulate a balanced homemade diet for our cats. There are several nutrients found only in meat and organs that the cat must get from the diet and are the key to its status as an obligatory carnivore. When we create our feline diet, we need to provide the following very specific nutrients that other carnivores, such as dogs, meerkats, raccoons, and bears, do not require.

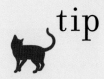
tip

Cats Are not Vegetarians

If you are vegan and you want a vegetarian animal companion you can feed according to your personal philosophy, get a rabbit, rodent, bird, or goldfish— but definitely not a cat. If you want to share your life and home with a cat, you must honor this "obligate carnivore" by feedingit according to its nature and needs. A non-meat-based diet is not appropriate for a cat. This method of feeding will leave the cat malnourished with no reserve to fight injury, stress, or disease.

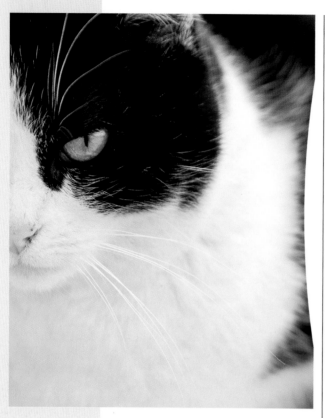

Black and White Domestic Shorthair

TAURINE

The amino acid taurine is essential for the health of cats' eyes, skin, and especially their hearts. We find taurine abundantly in their mother's milk and then in rich supply in muscles, eyes, and brain. The prey animal's heart is a muscle, this is a good source of taurine. Unlike dogs, cats cannot manufacture taurine from other amino acids, and they depend on a steady stream of it in their meaty meals. Taurine is not found in plants. Remember that the prey animal is the processing plant for many of the cat's nutritional needs. Pet food companies supplement with taurine, and we include taurine in our homemade recipe as well. Even though it is found in raw meat, it is so critical that we err on the side of safety. Before pet food manufacturers added it to their prepared foods, thousands of cats died of heart failure due to taurine deficiency. They found out the hard way that cooking destroyed taurine's bioavailability. Because taurine is found in between muscle cells, it is often lost in the meat grinding process as well.

ARGININE

Another amino acid essential for cats is arginine. Mammals use arginine in one pathway to metabolize ammonia, a toxic waste product of protein digestion. However, only the feline relies on arginine as its sole pathway for this reaction. A single low arginine meal will poison a cat on its own wastes, causing it to drool, stumble, and possibly seizure or die. Its mother's milk and meat are the cat's natural source of arginine.

VITAMIN A

Vitamin A is a feline requirement that can't be met by beta-carotene as it can in dogs. If you feed your cat carrots, he won't be able to get any vitamin A out of them. There is no pre-formed vitamin A in carrots; only beta-carotene, which cats cannot convert. Cats get their vitamin A needs met through their processing plant, the prey animal. The prey's liver is a rich source of pre-formed vitamin A, as is cod liver oil. (See Resources on page 174.)

VITAMIN D

People can turn precursors into biologically active vitamin D via the skin when it is exposed to sunlight. Cats love to spend hours laying in the sun, but they do not get any vitamin D this way because they do not have the right enzymes in their skin. The prey animal's liver is the cats' natural source of vitamin D. It is also found in cod liver oil.

NIACIN

Niacin, also known as vitamin B3, plays many roles throughout the body, including production of hydrochloric acid, formation of red blood cells, and generation of energy from foods. Most animals can make niacin in their own bodies from tryptophan, which we find in meat and the mother cat's milk. Cats have a very high need for niacin; they cannot create enough on their own and must consume it daily.

ARACHADONIC ACID

A fatty acid essential for cats, arachadonic acid plays an important role in maintaining healthy skin and coat. It's critical in reproduction and in healthy kidney function. Most animals can convert linoleic acid, which is found in animal fats and healthy oils, into arachadonic acid. Cats cannot manufacture arachadonic acid, which they primarily get from organ meats, such as heart, liver, and kidney. Cooking meat degrades arachadonic acid.

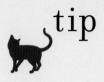
tip

How To Shop Raw

We recommend purchasing pasture raised or naturally raised, organic meat/poultry, and oil from wild-caught fish such as sardines or cod. Organic is especially important when feeding raw liver, as the liver is the body's major detoxification pathway, and contaminants can accumulate there. However, if the choice comes to store-bought meat or dry cat food, opt for meats that you would at least eat yourself!

See "Supplements and Whole Food Products" in Resources on page 174 for our favorite products and resources.

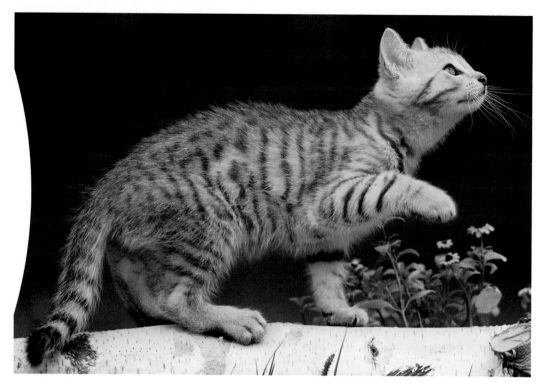

The tabby pattern naturally evolved into camouflage for cats in the wild.

LOVE AS THE MISSING INGREDIENT IN YOUR CAT'S FOOD

When we add love as an ingredient while making our cats' food, we are actually doing something quite scientific. A series of experiments studied rabbits that were fed a high-cholesterol diet intended to cause atherosclerosis (hardening of the arteries, which contributes to high blood pressure and heart disease). One group of rabbits received standard lab animal care (fresh food and water but minimal handling) while another group received daily visits from an experimenter who petted, handled, played with, and talked to the rabbits, essentially making them pets. The pet rabbits, who ate the same food as the other experimental rabbits—and whose blood cholesterol levels, heart rate, and blood pressure were also the same—had 60 percent less damage to their arteries.

Shopping for and preparing your cat's meals is a very loving and nurturing act. Cats can watch this preparation with anticipation. Serve cats their meals in a peaceful manner.

I recommend that you do not feed your cat (or eat your own meals) when he or you are stressed. Acute stress releases adrenaline, which shuts down the digestive system. When anxiety accompanies a meal, your food cannnot be properly digested, so nutrients can't get into your cells and function properly. This can compromise the immune system, making you vulnerable to infection and degenerative disease. All of our digestive functions work best when conditions are pleasurable. It's a double-edged sword for you, the caretaker of your family and pets. You must not only set the table, you must set the tone for meal time. Start with a smile. Don't let the kids or the dog interrupt. Turn on some classical music, but not too loud. It is within your control to set the stage for a peaceful mealtime. Put yourself in a loving mood, and be grateful to share your life with the amazing cat!

THE RAW FACTOR: AN ESSENTIAL COMPONENT IN YOUR CAT'S FOOD

Many people become very squeamish when they first hear about feeding raw meat. Remember that this would be the cat's choice in the wild. Now that cats live with us in our homes, we have removed that choice and forced them to eat things they would never find in the natural world.

Bacteria and parasites found in raw meat mandate safe meat handling procedures (by humans). The cat itself has many natural defenses. First, saliva contains an enzyme called lysozyme that attacks bacteria and other pathogens as the meat enters their mouth.

After this, any remaining contaminants must pass through the cat's extremely acidic stomach where the vast majority of bacteria are killed. The cat's short small intestine pushes food through quickly so invaders cannot get a foothold. (The cat's body length-to-digestive tract ratio is only 1:4, compared to 1:6 for the dog and human, 1:12 for the horse, and 1:20 for the cow.)

Finally, the undigested portion of the food passes through the large intestine, where competition from normal resident bacteria protects against invaders. These defenses destroy approximately 98 percent of bacteria such as *Salmonella*.

Freezing raw meat for seventy-two hours at 24°F (-4°C) kills protozoal parasites such as *Toxoplasma* (which humans are much more likely to contract from eating undercooked meat or gardening).

While it's true that bacteria aren't affected by freezing, consider that a mother cat licks the backsides of her kittens, and she ingests what comes out of them for several weeks following their birth. Cats clean their own bacteria-laden backsides and bodies for the rest of their lives, so you can appreciate the natural cleansing ability of the cat. However, depending on the health of your cat, you should proceed cautiously to introduce a homemade diet. You may need to begin by cooking the meat

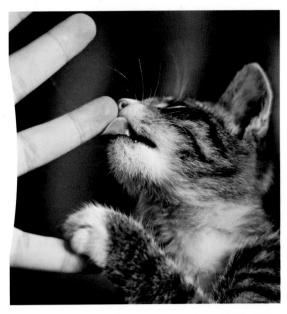

Domestic Shorthair

for very sick animals. Over time, you can cook the meat less and less until you're feeding it completely raw. The road to wellness and recovery will depend on shifting the cat's diet as close to nature as possible.

The *raw* aspect of the cat's natural prey diet is so critical that we must consider it to be an essential component of the diet. When we feed our cats a fresh or fresh frozen homemade meal with raw meat as its number one ingredient, their intestinal tracts remain healthy and strong. In fact, when the cat is fed its species-specific raw diet, it is healthier and thus more resistant to all diseases.

Inspired by Pottenger's Cats

A highly controversial series of studies, informally known as Pottenger's Cats, was done between 1932 and 1942 on the subject of raw vs. cooked foods for cats. Francis M. Pottenger Jr., M.D., conducted this experiment over many generations of cats to determine the effects of cooked food on their health. The group of cats that were fed cooked foods failed to thrive. Today's modern pet food scientists largely discredit this study, blaming the fact that cooking alters the bioavailability of taurine for the failure to thrive by the cooked food group. Indeed, many of the problems, including reproductive failure, poor growth, and heart problems, can be attributed to taurine deficiency. However, taurine alone does not account for all the changes discovered in Dr. Pottenger's research, such as bone and dental abnormalities, allergies, hypothyroidism, lung disease, and impaired immunity resulting in infections and parasitic infestations.

Dr. Pottenger fed various combinations of raw or cooked meat, raw or evaporated or pasteurized milk, and cod liver oil to different groups of cats. The cats that ate cooked meat rapidly declined in health, and it took several generations before their descendents truly regained their health.

These studies inspired me to create my raw homemade diet and supplements, which I've now fed to eleven healthy generations of Tonkinese cats. The results of this personal experiment have become my life's work. Once I read Pottenger's studies (I urge you to, as well) and viewed the original film *Pottenger's Cats* on DVD, I could not open another bag or can. The benefits of feeding raw meat were so numerous that they allayed my fears of the concept of raw meat. We've all been told that it is dangerous to handle, let alone eat. When I speak before crowds at cat shows, for example, I often ask, "What is a cat's natural diet?" They look at each other and are stumped for an answer. I then say, "Doesn't anybody watch *Wild Kingdom*?" "Oh," they say, "Those are wild cats. Aren't cats today different?" The correct answer is, "No, they are not!" Physiologically, dogs are wolves, and cats are tigers. It's as simple as that.

In Pottenger's Cats, as the feeding experiments were completed and the cats were removed from their pens, weeds began to sprout. There were noticeable differences in the size and health of these weeds, and the weeds grew better in the pens where the cats that had been fed raw food lived compared with where the cooked-food-fed cats lived. This further demonstrated the direct relationship between the health and vigor of the animals that lived in these pens and the excrement that fertilized the soil. Healthful eating had a ripple effect in the entire ecology!

Cat Fanciers' Association's Grand Premier Celestecats Macadamia, Platinum Mink Tonkinese, fourth generation raw food–fed cat.

People feed their cats in many different ways—some better, others not so good. To help you understand how your current feeding practices affect your cat's health, we'll rank each regime by a "paw" system. The best, healthiest food gets a five-paws rating, while the least healthful and nutritious gets only one paw. Any of these methods will fall somewhat short of the diet that the wild cat catches himself, but obviously that method of feeding isn't practical—or safe, given the dangers of outdoor life.

Wherever you are in the "Paws System," do your best to achieve "five paws." Your cat depends on you to provide a healthy diet. It will be worth every bit of effort to avoid the many health problems associated with poor diets, and to help your cat heal from any problems he has or that may be brewing deep inside.

THE PAW SYSTEM: ASSESSING THE QUALITY OF YOUR CAT'S DIET

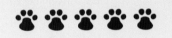	Raw meat-based homemade food (see our recipe on page 70) or commercial raw meat diets. (Health food and specialty pet food stores carry some brands, or you may also be able to find freeze-dried raw meat diets on the market. Try to find foods that have similar ingredients to the recipe on page 70.)
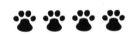	The same ingredients as five-paws food, but the food is lightly sautéed for a few minutes. This can be an intermediate stage in transitioning to raw. (You'll need to add extra taurine and digestive enzymes after the food has cooled to eating temperature.)
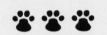	Organic or natural canned cat food: A sprinkle of digestive enzymes is a must. To take this diet up a notch, add a little raw or lightly cooked fresh meat to each meal, or whenever you can. Even a weekly treat of raw meat is far better than none.
	"Premium" and "super-premium" canned cat food from the giant, highly advertised manufacturers, such as the major brands at pet food retailers that are often sold by or recommended by veterinarians (Supplement the food with enzymes and essential fatty acids.) Grocery and discount store brand, generic, and private label canned foods. (Their ingredients tend to be of even poorer quality than the premium and super-premium foods.)
	Dry food (kibble): We highly recommended, for the quality of life and health of your cat, that you upgrade from a dry food diet. See "Switching Foods" on page 72 to get even the fussiest cat to eat a better diet.

A PROPERLY PREPARED HOMEMADE DIET

You may have decided to make your own cat food for all the reasons we have presented. You may have performed independent research or perused other books before reading this one. However, most diets and recipes found in pet "cookbooks" or online are not complete or balanced. Many veterinarians are absolutely against raw and homemade diets of any kind exactly because they have seen animals that have become very sick from improperly made homemade diets. The most serious problems arise from simply feeding raw meat as a substitute for commercial cat food. What the cat needs is a diet *based* on raw meat, but also containing supplements that provide all necessary nutrients, including calcium and other minerals, vitamins, healthy fats, enzymes, amino acids, and other trace nutrients. As we'll talk about next, feeding only raw chicken necks, backs, and wings is not a properly prepared raw meat diet.

NEWS FLASH: A CHICKEN IS NOT A MOUSE

Modern livestock and poultry contain a very unnatural meat-to-bone ratio. Meat animals have been bred to produce much more muscle and fat than a wild mouse, bird, or other natural feline prey. This must be taken into account in balancing your cat's diet, especially if you are using bone-in ground meat or poultry. We have calculated this for you in our recipe.

To illustrate this difference, here is a comparison of the nutrient content of a mouse versus a chicken bred for meatiness. Bone mineral content is the major component of "ash." As you can see, for the same calorie (gross energy) intake, the mouse has nearly twice as much ash, compared to protein, as the chicken.

NUTRITIONAL CONTENT OF MOUSE VS. DOMESTIC CHICKEN

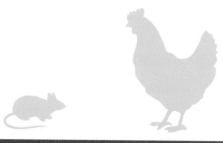

FIELD MOUSE	ADULT CHICKEN
32.7% Dry Matter	32.5% Dry Matter
55.8% Crude Protein	42.3% Crude Protein
23.7% Crude Fat	37.8% Crude Fat
11.8% Ash	9.4% Ash
5.25 Kcal/g Gross energy	5.9 Kcal/g Gross energy

Many people start out with a decent recipe and the best intentions, but over time they run out of a supplement and forget to replace it, or they get in the habit of feeding just one kind of meat, or they get off the track in some way or another. As with humans, this is called "diet drift." It is one of the easiest ways to create nutritional deficiencies or excesses—and consequently serious health problems—for your cat.

THE WRONG RAW DIET

To illustrate how a raw-food diet with the best intentions could go awry, consider the case of Safari. Safari was a one-year-old exotic Serval cat (*Felis serval*) when he came to live with his human mom, an exotic rescue professional. He was very ill at the time. Every morning, Safari vomited yellow bile, and he had failed to thrive. The vet had Safari eating a meat-only diet with the bone in, as commonly, but wrongly, advocated in many books and websites.

Safari's caregiver sent me his blood work, which I analyzed from a clinical nutrition standpoint. I decided to revamp this all-meat–and-bone diet. I recommend adding some sweet potato (yam) to raw beef or chicken, our special vitamin/mineral powder, our essential fatty acid blend, and our digestive enzyme supplement, turkey heart, and other organ meats. Safari wasn't keen on the mixture at first, so I suggested adding some canned wild Alaskan red salmon for flavor. He liked it and dove right in. At the time he began his new diet, the vomiting had occurred every morning, regardless of whether he had eaten or not. In a matter of days after Safari started his new regime, the vomiting stopped.

It is our experience that a diet of strictly feeding chicken necks, backs, or wings or turkey necks, as so many advise, is extremely harmful. It's too much bone, and it lacks many vitamins and minerals. The exotic cat diet, like that of domestic cats, must be properly balanced and supplemented.

Safari, now thirteen years young, gets a diet consisting of raw meat and yam in the morning, two frozen chicks in the afternoon, and a few times per week he has turkey hearts in his food and a turkey neck for dessert. Safari's owner grows pots of cat grass for him that he loves to nibble on after dinner. Perhaps that's because Safari's cousins still roam the savannahs and forests of Africa, where they naturally chew on grass. We can provide the same experience for our cats by growing organic grass seeds selected especially for cats.

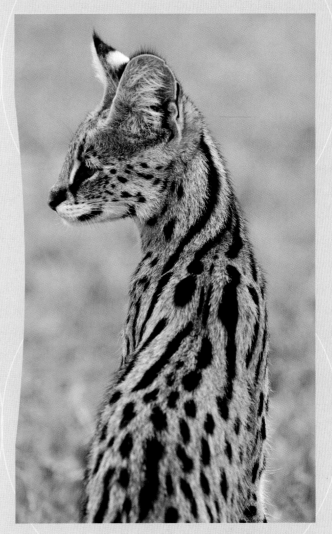

Felis serval *in the wild*

BASIC FRESH RAW FOOD RECIPE

It is so important to use common sense when feeding your cat a homemade raw meat diet. Some cats also enjoy small amounts of vegetables, while others resist them. You'll just need to experiment on your own little tigers to see which way they prefer.

YIELD.

Approximately two to four days worth of food for an average ten-pound (4.5 k) adult cat. Increase for kittens and pregnant or lactating queens.

INGREDIENTS

- 1 lb. (0.45 kg) raw coarse ground, minced, or diced beef or poultry, up to 20 to 25 percent fat (Do not use pork or fish; limit ground lamb due to its high fat content.) Try venison, elk, bison, ostrich, quail, and other poultry, and alternate and/or combine meats for variety.

- ¼ lb. (100 g) raw minced or diced organic organ meat, such as liver, kidney, heart, and gizzard (turkey, chicken, beef, or lamb).

- 8 ounces (250 ml) purified water combined with 4 drops of grapefruit seed extract (GSE) liquid concentrate.

- 2 level tablespoons (20 g) feline supplement for a homemade raw meat diet (use manufacturer's recommended amount), such as Celestial Cats Vitamin/ Mineral+ Feline (VM+) Supplement. Note: Cut the amount of Celestial Cats VM+ in half if using bone-in ground meat.

- 2 tablespoons (30 ml) Celestial Cats Essential Fatty Acid (EFA) Oil Blend and/or 1 tablespoon (15 ml) pharmaceutical grade omega-3 fish oil supplement such as Nordic Naturals Cod Liver Oil, plus 100 IU vitamin E.

- 1 drop liquid garlic extract such as Kyolic Aged Garlic Extract. (Too much garlic can cause serious health consequences. Do not oversupplement and never use raw garlic.)

- ⅛ to ¼ teaspoon Celestial Cats Feline Enzyme Supplement.

- 500 milligrams taurine (powder or capsule).

OPTIONAL INGREDIENTS

- 2 to 4 ounces (60 to 120 g) food-processed raw zucchini (or pureed steamed), food-processed or pulped raw or baked yams, canned organic unsweetened pumpkin, or organic baby food vegetables such as sweet potatoes (yams), carrots, or winter squash. (No corn or potatoes.)

(See "Supplements and Whole Food Products" in Resources on page 176 for suppliers of the supplements mentioned in this recipe.)

Refrigerate EFA oil, cod liver oil, and Kyolic garlic after opening.

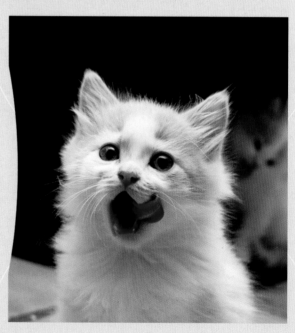

Domestic Longhair kitten

PREPARATION

1. Because *all* whole bones (including vertebrae) can splinter, you can have your butcher grind chicken backs and necks—or even a whole chicken. Be sure the butcher runs them through the grinder at least three times. You could also purchase your own meat grinder and grind your own meats and poultry. You may use a mallet to crush whole chicken necks and cut into thirds as "dessert" (feed only on a full stomach).

2. Treat the meat/poultry with the purified water/ grapefruit seed extract liquid concentrate. Note: Never use grapefruit seed extract straight (internally or externally). It will cause serious chemical burns. It must always be properly diluted. Place the meat in a bowl and pour the liquid over it in small amounts, blending it into the meat as you go. Use only enough of this solution necessary to make the food the consistency of a thick chili. (Alternatively, you could let the meat defrost in this solution in the refrigerator and do not drain off.)

3. Cut the organ meats and any other larger pieces of meat into bite-size chunks. Liver can be cut partially frozen and cut into cat size bites. Chicken necks can marinate in this solution as well rendering them a little softer. Cut up the chicken fat from the necks and use in the food if more fat is needed.

4. Mix all ingredients.

RAW FOOD RECIPE NOTES

- If you are just starting your cat on raw food, follow the guidelines on switching foods on page 72. Increase portions or feed more small meals if your cat gobbles it all up and wants more; amounts can vary from meal to meal. Do not overfeed.

- Leave food down for approximately an hour. If it's too warm in your home, or if flies are a problem, shorten the time. Unrefrigerated food spoils quickly.

- Feed on flat plates (cats hate to have their whiskers touch the side of a bowl) and let them eat at their convenience in peace. If they walk away, so be it. They'll be back in a few minutes.

- If organ meat is difficult to obtain, include a variety of gland and organ concentrates. (See "Supplements and Whole Food Products" in Resources on page 174 for suppliers.) Note: the Celestial Cats VM+ contains glandular and organ powder, so concentrates are not needed when using this product.

- Cats and kittens want their food very fresh. Therefore, keep food in the refrigerator for no more than three days. Store the food in glass bowls with tight lids. Plastic off-gasses organo-chlorines, which are toxic to people and pets. (See "Miscellaneous Products" in Resources on page 176 for companies that sell these bowls.)

- Always defrost meat in the refrigerator—never in the microwave. (See "Microwave Ovens" on page 50.) Safe handling of raw meat is imperative. Wash hands, dishes, and utensils in hot soapy water. Clean surfaces with environmentally safe cleaning products, such as a solution of 1 drop of grapefruit seed extract per ounce (30 ml) of water.

- Try to use a supplement designed for a homemade diet, such as the Celestial Cats supplements, which were specifically designed for this recipe and tested on eleven generations of the Celestecats Tonkinese Cats. The supplement should include correct proportions of bone meal, super greens, and gland and organ powder to balance the recipe properly.

- Most importantly, serve with love. Please check with your holistic practitioner before changing your cat's diet, as any change can be stressful.

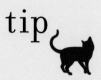

tip

Starting Kittens on the Raw Diet

Kittens are introduced to solid food at five weeks old, starting with ½ to 1 teaspoon (2.5 to 5g) per kitten, four to six times a day, while they are still nursing. Some kittens eat with mom and do just fine so long as several meals a day are provided. Increase amounts to approximately 2 tablespoons (30 mls) per kitten as they grow. After twelve weeks, feed three to four times daily. After six to eight months of age, they may cut back on feedings themselves. Some cats will always prefer three meals per day, but after one year of age, most cats can be fed twice a day. Cats and kittens reach their proper weight on this diet when fed according to their needs.

OVERCOMING RAW-FOOD DIET OBSTACLES

In spite of the simple recipe provided on page 70, preparing your cat's food at home may seem too big a challenge for many reasons. The two most common objections relate to *time* and *money*.

IT TAKES TOO MUCH TIME. Many people who are new to this method of feeding worry about how time-consuming the preparation of homemade meals may be. All you need is a system. For instance, make large batches and freeze in meal-size portions.

IT'S TOO EXPENSIVE. The initial expenses of a homemade diet can be daunting. You need to buy supplements, and you may want to invest in tools, such as a meat grinder or food processor, to make the job easier. Remember, a raw food diet is the ultimate preventative health measure. It is a virtual certainty that your cat will develop one or more chronic diseases on a commercially prepared diet. A species-specific diet will save you money on veterinary bills in the long run.

SWITCHING FOODS

Many cats and kittens immediately love their new raw food diet. It's a good sign to have a cat with a hearty appetite. But for others it takes a bit of strategy to accomplish this goal. Here are some tips for making this transition. For cats who have had food available day and night (free choice), the first step is to go to a timed meal schedule, where you leave the food out for an hour in the morning and again for an hour in the evening, but put it away the rest of the time. Believe me, your cat will not starve to death in twelve hours. The eat-fast-eat schedule is more natural to carnivores, and it gives them time to digest between meals. Also with this schedule, you don't have to worry about restricting the amounts you feed; the cat will eventually self-regulate very well on this schedule. The other big advantage of timed meals is that your cat will be hungry at mealtime, and thus more willing to try new things. This is particularly critical when switching from dry food.

Many people have tried—and failed—to convert their cats to better diets. A primary reason for that is the tendency of cats to turn their noses up at any new food. Most cats' food preferences were formed during kittenhood. In fact, many cats who have been fed only dry food their whole lives simply don't recognize anything else as "food." Getting a food-addicted cat just to change brands or flavors can be a major challenge. Cats often require a more gradual (that is, sneaky) approach, with several intermediate stages over weeks or even months. Cats dislike change in general, and messing with their dinner habits may not be welcome. But it is almost always possible to convert cats to a better diet.

When adding raw food, or switching from dry to canned or raw, use caution and go slowly. These forms of food are so vastly different that it will take some serious getting used to on the part of your cat's tummy. If your cat eats dry food, it may be easier to switch to any canned food first, and then move to a better canned food and ultimately raw. Just getting a dry-food addict to eat a good quality canned food is a very worthwhile improvement and a good first step! Start with just a tiny amount, perhaps a teaspoon, of canned food mixed into the dry food. Work up to 25 percent wet food, then 50-50, then 75-25. With the last 25 percent, introduce the raw food recipe and increase the raw ration incrementally. Be sure to add digestive enzymes if using any cooked or processed foods.

If your cat refuses dry with canned or raw mixed in, offer only the new food for the first half of the meal period before offering the cat her normal food. Many cats will be hungry enough to at least taste it. (When dry food gets wet, surface bacteria will rapidly grow; discard leftovers not eaten within the meal period.)

If you're having trouble switching your cat's food, try one of the following tricks.

🐾 Start with plain meat, without veggies or supplements.

🐾 Lightly brown the meat before serving.

🐾 For dry food addicts, sprinkle a handful of kibble on top of canned or raw food.

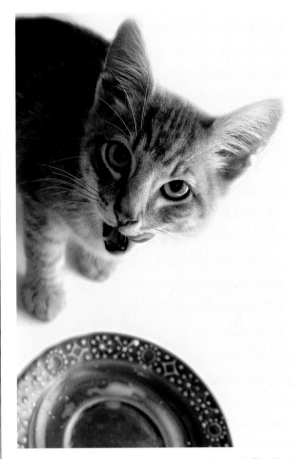

Domestic Shorthair

🐾 Crush the dry food into crumbs. Make tiny, bite-sized meatballs of the new food and roll them in the crumbs.

🐾 Incorporate a bribe food, such as canned salmon, sardines, or mackerel; their rich smell is irresistible to many cats.

🐾 Spread chicken or turkey baby food on top of the food. (Make sure the baby food does not contain onion powder, which is toxic to cats, or cornstarch, which is potentially allergenic.)

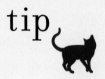

tip

Why Food Enzymes Are Essential

Food enzymes are as essential for cats as they are for all mammals. There are thousands of enzymes in every living cell, some of which are digestive enzymes. The cat's natural diet of raw prey takes advantage of these enzymes to aid its own digestion. Cooking and processing of food destroys (denatures) these vital enzymes. Without them, the cat's pancreas must secrete more of its own enzymes to compensate. Such artificially created stress is a precursor to a great number of chronic and acute health problems. (Cooking also reduces the water content and alters the protein structure of the meat, making it more difficult to digest.)

A balanced enzyme product (containing amylase, cellulase, lipase, and protease) must always be added to any cooked cat food product to help the cat digest its food thoroughly and get the maximum benefit from the nutrients. Enzymes are also used with the raw homemade diet as well, especially if raw food-processed vegetables are included. This is because in the wild, the cat would obtain this vegetable matter predigested in the prey animals' gastrointestinal tract, where digestive enzymes would have already done their job. Wild cats eat the entire kill from head to tail!

Processed commercial pet foods are a long way from fresh, raw foods containing their own enzymes. Because of this, part of the digestive process for dry food is putrefaction (rotting). It takes up to twenty-four hours for dry food to pass through the cat's approximately 4 foot (1.2 m) intestinal tract and eight to ten hours for cooked or canned foods. Raw food transits the cat's system in approximately four hours, making its first appearance in the small intestine in twenty minutes. Digestive enzymes make the transition easier, although a raw diet is usually the easiest to digest. Often times cats regurgitate the new food because they have eaten too much at once. A wild mouse is less than two tablespoons (30 g) worth of food.

Always make sure your cat is eating at least half of her normal intake at each meal. If not, take a step backward in terms of percentages, or offer your cat's favorite food by itself. Cats (especially overweight cats) can quickly develop hepatic lipidosis (fatty liver disease) if they eat too little or miss even a few meals. Lipidosis is expensive to treat, and not all cats survive. Watch out for loss of appetite, which is both a cause and a symptom. Sometimes cats with lipidosis vomit. If lipidosis progresses, cats lose weight and become jaundiced. (Their skin and the whites of their eyes turn yellow.)

Many (if not most) cats will have a change in stool, even diarrhea, with a change of diet. As long as the cat is still eating well and acting fine, mild diarrhea is normal, even if it persists for a week or two. (Caution: If your cat has additional symptoms, such as lethargy, poor appetite, or persistent vomiting, stop the new food and contact your veterinarian.)

Here are some ways to prevent or resolve diarrhea due to diet change.

- Make the switch very slowly or decrease the amount of new food being fed and go back to a larger proportion of the old food.

- Temporarily (for up to 2 weeks) switch to plain boiled chicken with canned pumpkin, cooked basmati rice, or rice baby cereal. Add digestive enzymes but no other supplements. Use this as the basis for your switch to raw, instead of going back to the previous diet.

- Add a digestive enzyme supplement. Enzymes should be plant- or fungal-based (not pancreas extracts) and include protease, lipase, amylase, and cellulase. (See "Supplements and Whole Food Products" in Resources on page 174 for some suppliers.)

- Add probiotics to help balance the gut's bacterial population. Probiotics are "friendly" bacteria such as *Lactobacillus acidophilus* and *Bifidobacterium bifidum*. (See "Supplements and Whole Food Products" in Resources on page 174 for recommended suppliers.)

Fasting When Ill

Most animals, but especially cats, will naturally fast when they are ill. Skipping one or two meals isn't cause for alarm as long as there are no other serious symptoms. However, many people recommend force-fasting cats periodically—sometimes as often as once a week. For a truly healthy cat, this wouldn't pose a problem, but it isn't a natural behavior unless they're sick. For the cat who is not in optimum health, fasting can be dangerous. It can trigger the liver to shut down, which can be fatal. We do not recommend involuntary fasting.

STIMULATING THE APPETITE

A piece of a sardine in chicken broth is helpful for cats who are ill, especially those who are suffering from upper respiratory infections. When a cat or kitten's nose is stuffed up, she can't smell her food, and if she can't smell her food, she will not eat. Something strong smelling such as sardines, jack mackerel, or canned wild salmon, in chicken broth will encourage her to eat. (Caution: Some commercial chicken broth, even organic, contains onion, which is toxic to cats.)

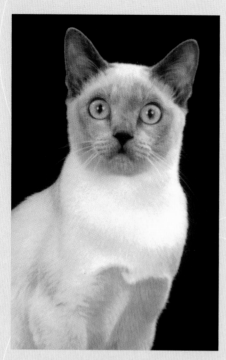

The International Cat Association's Grand Champion Celestecats Satin Doll, Blue Point Tonkinese, second generation raw food–fed cat

A Hard Lesson:

THE IMPORTANCE OF CALCIUM

Calcium deficiencies (in humans and animals alike) lead to nervousness, lameness, muscle spasms, heart palpitations, seizures, and of course bone fractures. Calcium allows us all to be able to think and even raise our arms/paws.

In the wild, cats eat the whole prey animal, including its bones. In nature, bones supply calcium. Meat consumed without bones or bone meal is very high in phosphorus, which must be properly balanced with calcium.

Natural feeding is at the heart of our breeding program, and we intend it to continue throughout the lifetime of the cat. A kitten in our program can go to its first show at four months of age, progress through shows and accumulate points and titles. At about one year of age, a cat may then enter the breeding program, where he or she will remain until the next generation is ready to take over. At that time, we retire them, spay or neuter them, and find them loving homes where we want them to be kept on my complete feeding regime. We review the diet, supplements, and holistic principles with each prospective new guardian. They sign contracts that state they will use their best efforts to continue with our regime. (They also agree not to declaw and to keep the cat indoors.) They leave with our complete starter kit: recipes, Celestial Cats supplements (See "Supplements and Whole Food Products" in Resources on page 176 for more information. Our supplements contain the best quality bone meal from New Zealand organic beef), some of our cat litter, premade food from the batch the cats are currently eating, and of course, full access to us for future assistance.

Unfortunately, we cannot always stay in touch with all adoptive parents. When we don't hear from a new guardian, we worry. When they don't return calls, we worry even more. (When their number has been disconnected, we feel sick to our stomachs.) One new owner had not returned our phone calls, and we had been out of touch for almost ten years. When we did hear from her, she wanted another cat just like her beloved girl, whom, she told us, had passed away. She explained that one day her kitty just couldn't get up, or even take another step if she was lifted to her feet. The guardian had been preparing the cat's raw food for years without our supplements, bonemeal, or bones in the diet. This meant there had been no calcium in the meals whatsoever—just meat and a small amount of vegetables. Without proper supplementation, bone meal, raw ground bone, or any source of calcium in her food, the cat virtually self-cannibalized calcium from her own bones and cells. When there was no more calcium to be had, her muscles and heart could no longer function, leading to collapse, inability of her muscles to contract, and ultimately death.

Now that I am winding down my personal involvement in the breeding of cats and passing the baton off to my partners, I have told this story here in the hopes that this sort of tragedy never happens again. Sadly, there are many case reports just like this in the veterinary literature.

CALCIUM AND THE QUEEN

Pregnant and nursing female cats have a higher requirement for all nutrients, including calcium, especially in the last part of pregnancy and while they are nursing the kittens. To make sure our queens are well-nourished, we simply feed more meals—four times a day or as much as they want.

Muscle cells use calcium to contract. During a long or difficult kitten delivery, a queen can use up so much calcium with her labor contractions that she will start to gulp or gag, with a sort of spasm in the throat. In these rare cases, we immediately administer calcium by mouth, or we have the vet administer calcium intravenously. During lactation, queens need a calcium-rich diet, so they are fed extra bones and as much food as they want.

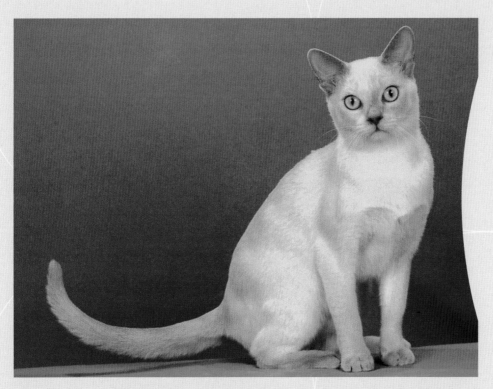

Cat Fanciers' Association's Grand Champion Celestecats American Beauty Rose, Distinguished Merit, Platinum Mink Tonkinese, fifth generation raw food–fed cat

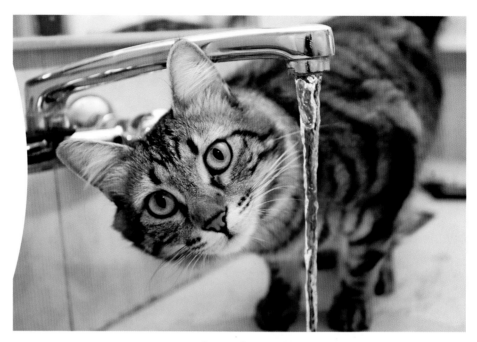

Cats are fascinated by running water—be sure it's purified!

THE IMPORTANCE OF PURE DRINKING WATER

Not all water is created equal. The kind of water your cat drinks can have a major impact on her health. Any water source can be filtered to make it healthier for your cat. The basic categories of water are: municipal tap water, well water, distilled water, and spring water. We'll talk about each in turn.

TAP WATER

The quality of tap water varies tremendously from one municipality to another. Municipal water generally contains chlorine, fluoride, and harmful contaminants such as bacteria, arsenic, toxic pesticide residues, heavy metals, and even rocket fuel. Some cities' water tastes bad, but taste is not a reliable indicator of what's really in there.

If you must use tap water, it should be filtered before your cat can safely drink it. Even a simple countertop filter will remove chlorine, lead, arsenic, bacteria, and some chemicals. Faucet-mount or canister filters are a step up; under-sink or whole-house filters are best. You'll find many brands and a huge variation in price, but in general, you get what you pay for. Reverse-osmosis filtered water should also have trace minerals added. (See "Water Resources" in Resources on page 174 for some suppliers.)

WELL WATER

Well water is sometimes pure and healthful, but other times it's full of bacteria, agricultural runoff, heavy metals, and other contaminants. The only way to be sure is to have the water tested. Again, filtration may be the best option if you are on well water.

DISTILLED WATER

Distilled water has been purified so that it does not contain any particles at all. While purity may sound good, you really should not use distilled water for drinking. Distilled water contains zero solutes, which are dissolved molecules, so when it enters the intestines, diffusion will actually pull solutes out of the body. Drinking only distilled water can ultimately cause deficiencies in sodium, potassium, and important trace minerals. While distilled water can be valuable when used for a short-term process of detoxification, it's not safe for long-term consumption unless you add trace minerals to it. (See "Water Resources," on page 174 and "Supplements and Whole Food Products" in Resources on pages 174 for suppliers.)

SPRING WATER

Spring water, if it's really from a natural spring and if the spring itself is good quality, is the best choice for cats—and the rest of the family, too! In general, avoid generic and grocery store brands because many of them test positive for bacteria and chemical contaminants, such as arsenic, chloroform, toluene, nitrates, and phthalates. Instead buy artesian spring water, which is purer because the layers of rock and clay around artesian aquifers provide protection from potential contamination.

You can provide the best food and great supplements for your cat, but if the water is poor quality, optimal health will remain out of reach. Pure, good quality water is an essential ingredient of your cat's wellness program.

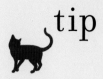
tip

Dr. Jean Learns About Tap Water the Hard Way

I realized the power of water years ago when I had to go out of town for a few days. My cat Marcus, who had Addison's disease, stayed at our clinic while I was gone. He ate only the raw diet I provided, but I didn't think about the fact that he would be given Denver tap water, which he never got at home because we had a faucet-mounted filter. Marcus developed severe vomiting and diarrhea while at the clinic, both of which cleared up immediately when I got him home and back on his own water. Since then I have seen many significant health improvements when cats stop drinking tap water. It's worth investing in a good water filter to provide pure water for your cat—as well as his human family!

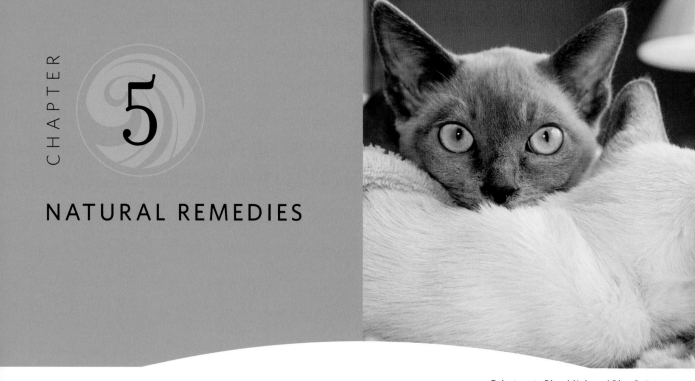

CHAPTER 5

NATURAL REMEDIES

*Celestecats Blue Mink and Blue Point,
sixth generation raw food-fed Tonkinese kittens*

The first step in holistic healing is to clean up the cat's lifestyle. That means feeding a wholesome, nutritious diet of fresh foods without all the processing and additives of commercial pet foods. Fresh food, fresh air, deep restful sleep, sunshine, and exercise are all essential for cats as much as they are for us. They give the body what it needs to heal itself.

Beyond diet and lifestyle changes, many cats will need extra help to reach a true state of health. In this chapter, you'll learn about some of the modalities used in veterinary medicine that can accelerate the healing process for your cat.

DETOXIFICATION

As you begin to make changes in your cat's diet and environment to remove the residue and effects of drugs, vaccines, anesthesia, chemicals, processed pet food, and infectious agents, the cat will go through a healing process called detoxification—detox. All natural healing substances and holistic therapies—including herbs, supplements, homeopathy, nosodes, flower essences, acupuncture, and aromatherapy—elicit a detoxification response. In this natural phase of the healing process, things may seem to get worse for a time, even though the body is actually moving forward to restore health and balance.

THE NATURE OF SYMPTOMS

Symptoms are simply the visible manifestation of the body's attempt to heal itself. For instance, when a virus infects the upper respiratory system, the body produces lots of mucus and tears to wash away the virus particles. Inflammation flares as the body's defensive white blood cells rush to the area and release chemicals to kill the invaders. Coughing develops as airway defenses push virus particles and debris away from the lungs. The cat may even develop a fever, since respiratory viruses cannot live at higher-than-normal temperatures. These symptoms may be uncomfortable for the cat, and certainly distressing for you to see, but they are all part of the normal defensive and healing processes of the body.

If, however, you give the cat drugs to suppress the symptoms, these normal defenses will be inhibited. The body then has to find another way to combat the infection, which often results in a new symptom. For instance, if a decongestant is used to dry up the mucus and tears, the virus may be able to penetrate deeper into the lungs, and a cough may develop to protect sensitive lung tissues. If we then use another drug to get rid of the new symptom—the cough—the body will continue to search for other ways to deal with the problem. For example, if a cough suppressant is given at this point, inflammation may develop in the lungs that can lead to pneumonia or even asthma.

To return the system to a normal, healthy state, whatever caused the problem in the first place must first be dealt with. In this case, the virus must be killed, and cellular debris resulting from the battle between the immune cells and the virus must be cleaned up and removed.

ENVIRONMENTAL CHALLENGES

The body—whether human or feline—receives constant challenges from the environment: viruses, bacteria, parasites, and fungi, and also air pollution, water pollution, and chemicals used in the manufacture of flooring, carpeting, furniture, and clothing. Because cats often sleep on rugs, sofas, and comforters, as well as walk on them and then lick their paws and fur, they take in far more toxins than humans. Cats' small body size and higher metabolic rate increase their intake and storage of these toxins.

Through the use of holistic therapies, accumulated toxins can be released by the cells and eliminated through the ears, eyes, and skin and through the respiratory, urinary, and digestive systems.

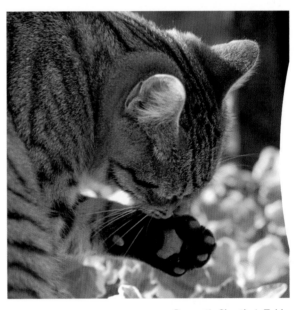

Domestic Shorthair Tabby

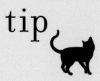

tip

How Can I Tell if My Cat's Symptoms are from Detox?

Common detox symptoms include mild vomiting and/or diarrhea, itchiness, skin rash, clear discharges from eyes or nose, sneezing, or symptoms related to problems your cat previously experienced. Symptoms that were originally suppressed by drugs or surgery may return for a short time as the body deals with them fully, which it was prevented from doing initially. (However, respiratory signs due to chronic *Herpesvirus* infection, are not necessarily from detox and may always persist to some extent.) If your cat, who eats normally and drinks water occasionally, suddenly stops doing either, take his temperature to be sure he's not running a fever. Use a digital rectal thermometer with a gel lubricant. The normal range for a cat is about 100° to 102°F (37.7° to 38.9°C).If your cat has a fever or is lethargic along with other symptoms, call your holistic veterinarian or natural health practitioner as soon as possible.

DETECTING AND TREATING DEHYDRATION

Healthy cats on a raw meat diet drink very little water, since they are designed to get the moisture they need from their prey. Cats eating dry food, as well as sick cats, drink water because they are dehydrated. When detoxing, the body often needs extra moisture to help flush toxins out of the tissues and into the excretory organs (kidneys, liver, digestive tract, skin, and lungs).

To test for dehydration, rub your finger along the cat's gums, which should be moist and slippery. If they are tacky or your finger sticks instead of slides, that's a sign of significant dehydration that must be treated with fluids.

If dehydration is serious, your veterinarian may need to use an intravenous catheter to rehydrate the cat, but in most cases, dehydration can be treated with subcutaneous fluids. You can administer subcutaneous veterinary fluids at home; ask your veterinarian or veterinary technician to give you a tutorial and provide you with the equipment and supplies required. Several websites offer detailed, visual instructions on this technique as well. (See Resources on Page 174 for more information.)

GIVING FLUIDS

Giving fluids is often the single most important thing you can do yourself to help your cat through an illness or a crisis. As long as your cat's energy and vitality are improving, the program is working. Whatever discharge or drainage you see is the result of the body cleansing itself and thus becoming healthier. However, as with all healing therapies, detox must be done gently to avoid dehydration or excess discomfort. For example, detox that causes a softened stool (the consistency of mashed potatoes) is a gentle cleanse, whereas diarrhea (brown or yellow water) may cause the patient to become dehydrated. If the cat clearly doesn't feel well, or the symptoms are worse than they were originally, the detox is too fast or too harsh. Stay in close touch with your practitioner so she can monitor your cat's progress and make sure that electrolytes and fluids stay balanced.

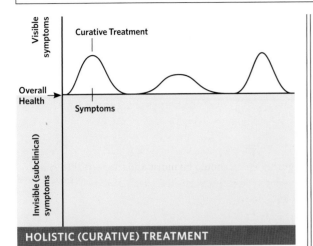

HOLISTIC (CURATIVE) TREATMENT

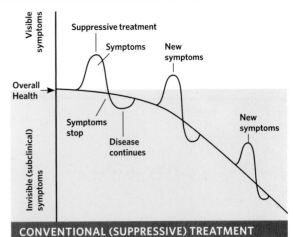

CONVENTIONAL (SUPPRESSIVE) TREATMENT

In this model, the animal begins with normal health. Symptoms appear, and appropriate holistic treatment that addresses the root cause is given. The disease is cured, and the animal's health returns to normal.

Administering suppressive treatment (such as antibiotics or anti-inflammatories) curbs the symptoms, but it does not cure the root cause. The disease remains active at a subclinical level (no visible symptoms). Over time, the disease is driven deeper into the system, and the animal grows sicker. Ultimately the disease reappears as something more serious or in a more vital organ. So, don't be surprised or alarmed if old symptoms return or even worsen during detox.

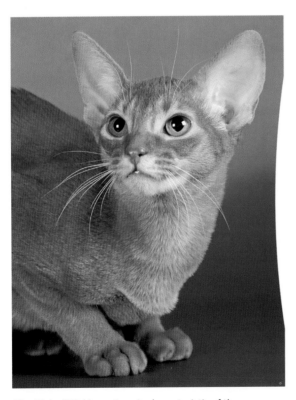

The "ticked" Tabby pattern is characteristic of the Abyssinian.

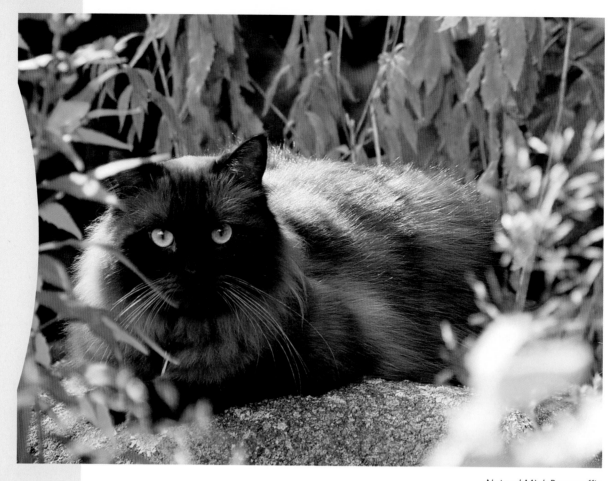

Natural Mink Ragamuffin

HERBS

The subject of herbs, like many of the healing therapies addressed in this book, cannot be covered completely in a single chapter. However, the information provided in this section offers an overview to start your foundational knowledge.

CAUTION:

Do not treat your cat with herbs by yourself. Herbs can be very powerful, and many are dangerous for cats, even some that are safe for people or dogs. It takes extensive knowledge and experience to use herbs for cats correctly. Cats are extremely sensitive and cannot detoxify many common herbal constituents. Always consult an experienced veterinary herbalist or a veterinarian familiar with herbs who can guide you responsibly. "Natural" does not necessarily equal "safe"!

A BRIEF HISTORY OF HERBALISM

Healing systems all over the world embrace herbalism. India is the home of 5,000-year old Ayurvedic medicine, a system of healing using foods, herbs, spices, and lifestyle modifications to balance the five elements (earth, air, fire, water, and ether) and the three doshas, or personality types (vata, pitta, and kapha) within an individual. Tibetans, whose medicine was under the control of Buddhist lamas and, therefore, closely linked to their religion, carefully coordinated the harvesting of herbs to coincide with helpful astrological influences. In the sixteenth century, Paracelsus, a Swiss physician and alchemist, popularized the ancient concept of the Doctrine of Signatures. This concept used the outward appearance of a plant to give healers an indication of what it could cure. For example, the seeds of nutmeg and walnuts resemble the brain, and thus were thought to improve mental abilities.

Traditional Chinese Medicine views disease as a sign of disharmony within the whole person. Herbs have been crucial to Chinese medical practitioners since about 2,500 B.C. Many of their formulas go back thousands of years, handed down through the generations in herbal dynasties. The five elements in Traditional Chinese Medicine—fire, earth, metal, water, and wood—form a network of relationships. Each element represents a season, a taste, an emotion, and parts of the body. For example, fire represents summer, bitter taste, joy, and the heart, small intestine, tongue, and blood vessels. The concepts of yang and yin and qi (or chi) complement the basic model of the five elements. Yang and yin represent balance, and qi represents vital energy.

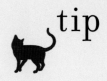

tip

Herbal Actions

Herbs are often classified by their actions or functions, and most herbs have more than one role to play in treatment. Here is a list of the most common herbal actions used in treating cats.

ADAPTOGEN: Increases vital energy, helps the body adapt to stress, supports normal functions, and restores functional balance to all organs and systems

ALTERATIVE: Gradually restores overall health

ANALGESIC: Relieves pain

ANTIEMETIC: Inhibits vomiting

ANTINEOPLASTIC: Inhibits tumors

ANTIOXIDANT: Destroys free radicals, which are a source of inflammation, degeneration, and aging

CATHARTIC: Laxative

FEBRIFUGE: Reduces fever

HEMOSTATIC: Stops bleeding

TONIC: Strengthens and invigorates

VULNERARY: Promotes wound healing

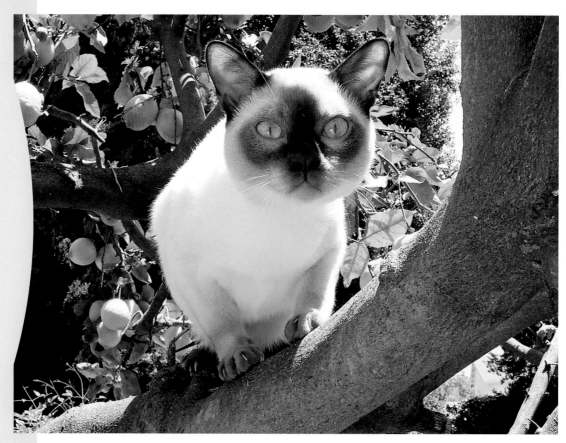

Cat Fancier's Association's Premier Celestecats Matrix, Champagne Point Tonkinese, sixth generation raw food-fed cat

HERBAL INGREDIENTS

Herbalists may use the bark, berries, bulbs, flowers, fruit, gum, hips, leaves, roots, root bark, seeds, tops, or the whole plant in a variety of traditions or recipes. Many modern drugs were first isolated from plants. For example, the salicylic acid in aspirin was isolated from the bark of the white willow tree, digitalis and digoxin are derived from the leaves of the foxglove plant, and taxol (a chemotherapy agent) comes from the bark of evergreen Pacific yew trees.

HERBAL PREPARATIONS

Herbs can be prepared in various ways, and the choice of method is often based on the toughness or fragility of the herb or whether its active ingredients are more soluble in water, alcohol, or oil. For instance, fragile flowers shouldn't be boiled because boiling will destroy their active components. The following preparation methods are those most commonly used for cats.

DECOCTION: A strong tea made from tough plants, roots, and bark. The herbs are boiled, and then steeped in pure water. This process extracts more minerals and bitter elements from the herb, but volatile elements can be lost.

INFUSION: A strong tea made from leaves or blossoms, made by pouring boiling water over the herbs and letting them steep. This process preserves the vitamins and volatile elements in fragile plants.

TINCTURE: An extraction of herbs in 100 percent alcohol. The finished tincture may contain 50 to 100 percent alcohol. Vinegar is sometimes used instead of alcohol.

EXTRACT: Extraction is a process of separating the active ingredients from the rest of the plant material. Extracts may be liquid (using water, alcohol, a water-alcohol mixture, or a water-vinegar mixture) or dry (evaporation or freeze-drying). Extracts are similar to tinctures but contain less alcohol (or vinegar).

POWDER: Dried herbs can be ground into a powder. The powder is typically manufactured into a tablet or capsule.

POULTICE: A moist, hot herb pack applied topically that can be used, for instance, to treat a bite wound or abscess. Fresh herbs should be crushed or mashed to release the active ingredients inside leaves or flowers. Powder is mixed with mineral water into a thick paste. Spread the poultice on a clean cloth and cover the affected area.

Many herbs suppress symptoms, just as many drugs do. This is not always the most desirable route to curing a disease, but it may be necessary for the comfort of the cat. Sometimes an herb is preferable to a similarly acting drug. But in other cases, the precise dosage or specific action of a drug may be required.

HOMEOPATHY

Homeopathy is a 200-year-old system of healing that uses remedies based on the Law of Similars, which is the reverse of the allopathic, or conventional, medical system. When used appropriately, homeopathy works with the body, not against it, promoting actual curing and not just suppressing symptoms. Homeopathic remedies stimulate the immune system, enabling it to complete the job it was already trying to do.

When in crisis, the human body, as well as that of the feline, speaks to us through its symptoms. Symptoms, produced by the body's attempt to heal, are windows to the internal process that should not be closed. All the symptoms, taken together, are referred to as the *symptomatic picture*.

LAW OF OPPOSITES, LAW OF SIMILARS

Allopathic, or conventional, medicine usually applies the Law of Opposites to the treatment of disease. The medication prescribed by the doctor or veterinarian acts *against* the patient's symptoms, as described by such names as *anti*biotic and *anti*-inflammatory. Allopathic drugs typically suppress symptoms but do not necessarily cure disease.

The Law of Similars means that the remedy that *causes* certain symptoms in a healthy person will *cure* the same symptoms in a sick person. For example, a bee sting (from the honeybee, *Apis mellifica*) causes an area of swelling and redness in normal individuals. The swelling may be accompanied by itching and burning, which feel better from the application of cold, and the person isn't thirsty. In homeopathic dilutions, the remedy *Apis mellifica* cures itchy, burning, red swellings that come on suddenly and are relieved by cold compresses, especially when the individual is less thirsty than usual.

The red swelling doesn't have to have been caused by a bee sting in order for *Apis mellifica* to be an effective remedy; it just needs to fit the same symptom picture. It may have been caused by something completely unrelated, such as sunburn, allergy, vaccinations, or drugs.

MINIMUM DOSE

Another main principle of homeopathy is the Minimum Dose. Homeopathic remedies are prepared by dilution and succussion, which is a particular way of mixing. They are so diluted that individual molecules of the original substance are extremely difficult to detect in samples. This allows remedies to be made from highly toxic substances, such as arsenic, snake venom, or the saliva of a rabid dog.

So, how does a remedy work if there virtually isn't anything there? When the mother remedy is made, the substance is mixed with water and succussed. This causes the water to receive an energetic imprint. Some might call it a ghost, a spirit, or even a memory. Science hasn't yet discovered or explained how homeopathy works.

The concept of minimum dose means that the more diluted the remedy is (in other words the less substance it actually contains), the more powerful it becomes, and the higher "potency" it is.

OUTCOMES OF HOMEOPATHIC TREATMENT

The principles of homeopathy state that there are three possible outcomes of any treatment: suppression, palliation, and cure.

SUPPRESSION rids the body of specific symptoms, but it drives the disease into other channels by denying the body's expression of the original disease. For example, a skin tumor develops that is itchy and eventually opens and drains. The allopathic vet may decide to remove the tumor and may not consider that this was the body's choice of a location to push toxins out. After surgery, the wound heals, and the skin looks great. The most troubling symptom is gone. Over time, however, the cat may experience a change in temperament (grouchier or more aggressive), or he may develop a more serious condition, such as thyroid disease or liver cancer. Since removing the original symptom, the cat has gotten very sick at a deeper level. It's like plugging the outlet of a volcano. It gets hotter and hotter inside until it explodes at a deeper, more dangerous level and causes much more destruction than it might have otherwise.

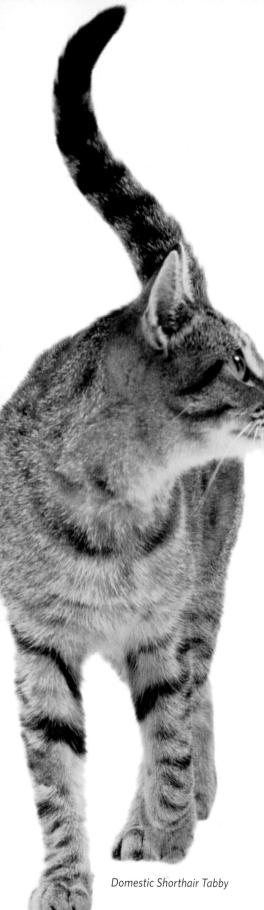

Domestic Shorthair Tabby

PALLIATION means to alleviate symptoms through medicine, such as treating pain through aspirin. With palliation, the medicine needs to be repeated frequently. Palliation makes symptoms go away almost immediately (even if they've been present or recurring for years). A cat may, for instance, temporarily stop crying when urinating, but the symptoms will soon return—in hours, days, or even far longer periods. Repeated dosing of a remedy, herb, or drug during palliation is a perpetual cycle to keep the symptoms away. The cat is not getting healthier and, in fact, is slowly getting sicker overall.

CURE, the goal of homeopathy, means that the body eliminates the whole disease, not just symptoms, and rises to a state of optimum health. Health is defined as not just the absence of symptoms, but a feeling of well being and vitality. A cure in classical homeopathy is more than just making the symptoms go away, which can happen with many kinds of treatments. Rather, it's when the symptoms go away and stay away permanently. The cat feels, and is, healthy in every respect. The cat may still get minor ailments, but recovers quickly from them with very little or no treatment.

By treating only symptoms and not the whole individual, allopathic, or conventional, medicine tends to be limited to the first two outcomes: suppression and palliation.

How Homeopathic Remedies Are Prepared

Today homeopathic remedies are still prepared according to guidelines given by Samuel Hahnemann, M.D., in *The Organon of the Healing Art* (1810). If possible, an alcohol tincture is made (some substances are not soluble in alcohol and are prepared differently). Dilution and succussion (shaking) of the tincture produce a *potentized* homeopathic remedy.

The level of dilution of a remedy is denoted with Roman numerals. One drop of the mother tincture diluted with nine drops of alcohol (or other solvent) creates a potency of 1X (as in X, the Roman numeral for ten). Similarly, 1 drop of the mother tincture diluted with 99 drops of alcohol creates a potency of 1C (as in C, the Roman numeral for 100). Higher potencies exist as well, such as M and LM. By the time a potency of 12C is reached, the dilution is beyond Avogadro's number (6.023×10^{23}, or 602,300,000,000,000,000,000,000,000), which in physical chemistry means that virtually nothing poisonous or toxic is left, no matter what the remedy has been made from.

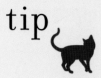

tip

Is a Cure Always Possible?

Through homeopathy, which most conventional veterinarians are not trained in, a real cure to most chronic diseases can be achieved in many cases where allopathic medicine offers only a quick (and often temporary) fix—if it has anything to offer at all. Homeopathy works particularly well for feline health problems, because cats are subtle creatures and highly sensitive to energy. Homeopathic remedies are easy to administer, and they encourage the body to help it heal itself.

If your cat has undergone long-term allopathic drug therapy, homeopathy may not work immediately. With persistence it may help restore the cat's health in cases in which conventional veterinarians might even recommend euthanasia. In the process of attempting a cure, very ill animals may at least feel better even if they can't be cured.

THE DEVELOPMENT OF HOMEOPATHY, HOMOTOXICOLOGY, AND HEILKUNST

HOMEOPATHY was developed by Samuel Hahnemann, M.D., a German physician, in the late eighteenth century. At that time, people were being treated with poisonous substances to get the "bad humours" out of them by making them vomit, have diarrhea, sweat, salivate, and bleed. Many patients died from these treatments.

Dr. Hahnemann felt such practices were barbaric, and he stopped practicing medicine. While making a living translating books, he came across William Cullen's write-up on the action of *Cinchona officinalis*, the herb used to make quinine for the treatment of malaria. Dr. Hahnemann disagreed with Cullen's assertion that it was the astringency of the herb that had the effect, and, to prove his point, took a small amount of the bark himself. He developed symptoms of malaria lasting a few hours. Dr. Hahnemann repeated the experiment several times, each time developing symptoms that went away by the next day.

From this research, Dr. Hahnemann developed the Law of Similars, derived from an ancient concept used by Galen, Hippocrates, and Paracelsus. When a healthy individual is made ill in a particular way by being exposed to a substance, that individual may also be cured by being treated with the same substance. Practitioners using Dr. Hahnemann's homeopathic system are called classical homeopaths.

HOMOTOXICOLOGY was developed by Hans Heinrich Reckeweg, M.D., a German physician who broke with traditional homeopathy to establish his own line of combination remedies—remedies that contained multiple homeopathics and/or multiple potencies. Each combination, however, is proven as a single remedy just like regular homeopathics. This form of therapy is also referred to as "biotherapeutics." (See Resources on page 174 for supplier information.)

HEILKUNST is a systematic approach to diet, nutrition, disease prevention, energetic immunization, and the removal of various diseases (everything from pathogenic to iatrogenic—drugs, vaccinations, and surgeries) that undermine the health of animals. Heilkunst uses Dr. Hahnemann's complete system, which encompasses not only homeopathy, but also diet, nutrition and lifestyle issues, energy and structural adjustments, detoxification and drainage, as well as an extensive disease classification and explanation system, involving natural, spiritual, acute, chronic, physical and mental diseases.

HOW A DISEASE RUNS ITS COURSE

In homeopathy, a cure is obtained by giving the substance whose experimental symptoms in healthy individuals are most similar to the patient's own symptoms. Since this therapy is based on an individual's total symptomatic picture, you must learn the characteristics of each remedy, observe carefully all the symptoms your cat is now exhibiting and has exhibited in the past, and understand her general characteristics.

Diseases tend to follow a predictable pattern. Here are the stages of disease:

ENERGETIC IMBALANCE: Your cat seems to be getting sick; there aren't any symptoms, but you just know something's wrong.

FUNCTIONAL CHANGES: For example, your cat is going frequently to the litter box, but there's no straining and the urinalysis is normal. If the disturbance is treated right away, even severe symptoms may resolve quickly or be avoided. At this point, a conventional veterinarian may not be able to diagnose the problem.

INFLAMMATION: If the disturbance remains untreated, inflammation shows that the body is trying its hardest to rebalance itself. At this stage the cat is sick, often with fever, redness, and swellings.

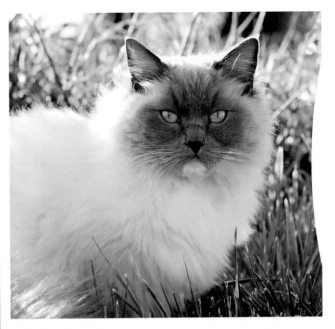

Blue Point Ragdoll

PATHOLOGY: Finally, the body tries to ward off the problem by moving into pathology, such as bladder stones; thick, hairless skin; or fluid accumulation in abdomen or chest. Once this stage has been reached, a cure takes longer to achieve. The cat must work her way back through the previous stages of the disease: inflammation, functional changes, and energetic imbalance. This is why it often seems as though the cat is worsening before improving. When a chronically ill cat is given an appropriate remedy, there will often be an immediate mental and emotional response of contentment, even though the final "physical" cure may take much longer.

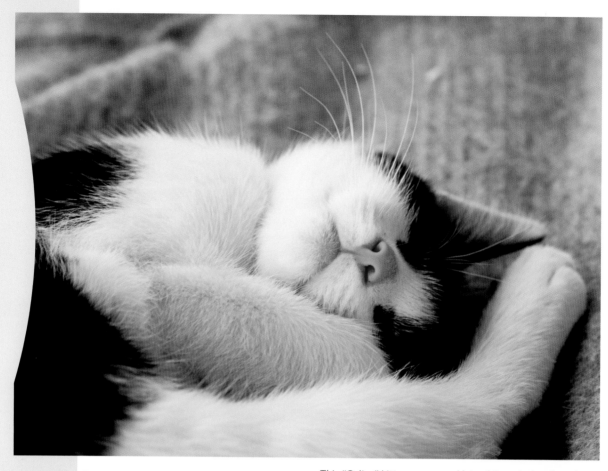

This "Calico" kitten may spend lots of time dozing, but always be observant to uncharacteristic changes in your cat's behavior.

WORKING WITH A HOMEOPATHIC PRACTITIONER

Never attempt to use homeopathy on your own to treat your cat. Always work with a homeopathic practitioner. Selecting the right remedy in the right potency at the right time is not a simple process, and assessing the progress of the case takes training and experience. Beginning homeopathic treatment seems expensive, but the costs are nearly all up front. Over time, you'll spend less money than you would have with conventional care and its repeated tests and treatments.

Your first appointment with a veterinary homeopath is likely to take an hour or more. He'll ask a lot of questions; some of which might seem irrelevant at first. In prescribing homeopathic remedies, the smallest details help the homeopath understand the cat's personality, which will help him distinguish among remedies. It is helpful for guardians to keep a journal of symptoms as homeopathic treatment progresses. Here are some questions to consider.

- How does your cat react to situations, people, other animals, noise, and other stimuli?

- Does your cat seek warmth under your covers or lie on the carpet or cool, hard surfaces?

- How much water does your cat drink?

- Does your cat like dry, soft, or soupy foods?

- How does your cat interact with other cats in the house?

- Is your cat the boss or the low cat on the totem pole?

A homeopath makes a list of all past and present symptoms, as well as of the individual's unique characteristics. The homeopath asks about every body system and what makes each symptom better or worse. He looks for changes in symptom pictures and tries to discover a cause for the changes (for example, symptoms started after the cat's human companions divorced). He also looks for characteristic symptoms (those symptoms that aren't normally associated with the disease). For example, everyone with the flu feels tired and achy, but characteristic symptoms might be feeling better from being consoled, worse from exposure to an open window, or better from having only cold drinks.

In many cases, this is the point where you and the cat will go home. Later, the homeopath looks up the most important and unique characteristics (and this takes experienced judgment) in a *repertory* containing tens of thousands of symptoms along with the remedies known to help each symptom. By cross-referencing the most important symptoms and traits, the homeopath comes up with the two to five best potential remedies.

Next, the homeopath compares his choices in a *materia medica*, which is a book containing in-depth descriptions of each remedy. He makes a selection and provides the remedy to you.

WAITING FOR A TRUE CURE

Be patient! A true cure takes time. Once a remedy is given, you must be vigilant about observing changes in the cat's symptoms, attitude, and any other signs or patterns the homeopath may ask you to watch. Keeping a journal is extremely helpful, noting observations and remedies along with the date, time of day, weather conditions, and any unusual stressors the cat has been exposed to. The homeopath will ask you to report back as things happen or at specified time periods; be sure to stick to the schedule.

The most common instruction you will hear from a classical homeopath is "Wait." Each remedy must be allowed to complete its work; for high potency remedies, a month or more is the minimum. Day-to-day changes should be noted in your journal, but try to see the bigger healing trends that are occurring. You will check in with the homeopath at intervals so that he can assess the case and make sure that the remedy is acting to cure, not to palliate or suppress.

When a homeopathic remedy is given, the energy field of the body immediately starts to react. In the first couple of days, the cat may seem to feel better, even if symptoms haven't changed. Three to five days after the remedy has been given, a response will usually be noticeable. This may look like current symptoms getting worse, older symptoms returning, or new symptoms arising—yet the cat clearly has better energy, a better appetite, or just looks more like his old self. An aggravation or healing crisis is a good sign; the body is being jolted into starting to heal itself. (Of course, if the symptoms get much worse and the cat is clearly feeling sicker, call your homeopath immediately for instructions; the remedy is not acting curatively and may need to be changed.)

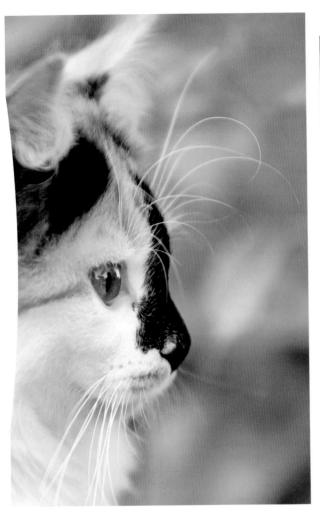

Calico Cat

When the aggravation or healing crisis occurs, it is critical to wait and not use another homeopathic remedy. You can make your cat more comfortable with other gentle treatments, such as massage, herbs, flower remedies, and Reiki.

Over time, the symptoms will slowly start to lessen. Again, the length of time needed for a cure is proportional to the length and depth of an illness and the amount of prior inappropriate treatment received, no matter if they were allopathic, homeopathic, herbal, or other. Cures take time and patience, and they often require several remedies over months or years. Patience is the key. If your cat is experiencing serious symptoms, such as difficulty breathing, you may need to get her emergency allopathic care, such as at a veterinary emergency facility. As soon as possible, let your homeopathic practitioner know what treatment the cat received . For example, if your cat develops a life-threatening asthma attack on Saturday, she might need steroids. But if you panic during a healing crisis with a cat already under homeopathic care and use allopathic treatment or give a homeopathic remedy on your own, you can create a difficult knot for your homeopath to untangle. It's challenging to decipher what requires emergency treatment and what is an acceptable level of crisis reaction. You should discuss this with your homeopath, but when the moment arrives, only you can make that decision.

It pays to be prepared, however. And homeopathy can be used to great advantage in first-aid situations for acute injuries or illness. You may want to keep a homeopathic kit on hand for emergencies in 30C potencies. Talk with your homeopathic practitioner in advance of an emergency to know how to use remedies properly. (See "Materia Medica" on page 96 for a list of the remedies to include in your emergency kit.)

Homeopathy is complex, and you can do serious harm with inappropriate remedies. Don't take chances with your precious cat's life. It's best to work with a veterinarian who is trained in small animal homeopathy, either in person or by phone, to select the right remedy, potency, and schedule of administration.

If you're seeking a homeopathic practitioner in addition to your conventional vet, be aware that many conventional veterinarians will welcome your search for another way to heal your cat. Other veterinarians may be threatened by new approaches, or feel they're not appropriate. Just be honest and, if you can, enroll them as your partner in healing.

DOSAGES

Homeopathic remedies are available in tablets and granules. Because the size of the animal isn't important, the dosage is the same for cats as it is for humans. The potency selected and how frequently it's given are more important than the amount given. If your cat doesn't swallow a complete dose (for example exactly three pellets), he'll still get the benefit. Your homeopath will help you determine a proper dosage schedule.

It's best to give homeopathic remedies on an empty stomach. However, if necessary, the remedy may be given in a small amount (approximately 1 teaspoon) of organic milk or cream or in wet food.

If your cat hates being pilled, it's easier to dissolve the remedy in water and administer it with an eyedropper. Here's how to make up a liquid remedy.

① Add the prescribed number of pellets or tablets to 1 ounce (28 ml) distilled water in a sterilized amber or cobalt glass dosage bottle. (Dark colored glass prevents light damage.).

② Shake the bottle vigorously against your hand one hundred times. This process is called succussing, and it helps distribute the remedy throughout the water. Pellets may take days to dissolve, but the remedy will be present in the water immediately.

③ Give a few drops by mouth.

No Expiration Date

Homeopathic remedies don't seem to lose their effectiveness unless they are stored improperly. Remedies one hundred years old have been used successfully! Just be sure to store your remedies away from sunlight, heat, strong odors, microwaves, motors, electrical equipment, and disinfecting agents.

Emergency First Aid

The materia medica and mini-repertory on the following pages are for first aid and informational purposes only. We do not advocate treating a chronic or serious disease without an experienced homeopathic practitioner. Remember that every remedy listed here may be used for many different conditions and that homeopathy treats the whole individual, not the problem.

The following remedies are excellent to have on hand for emergencies. Each remedy is listed by its full Latin name, although most also have an abbreviated name. For instance, *Aconitum napellus* is commonly referred to as *Aconite*, *Cinchona officinalis* is known as *China*, and *Silicea* is also called *Silica*.

Acute diseases and serious injuries often require higher potencies. Always consult your practitioner before administering remedies to pregnant or lactating cats.

Use a 30C potency unless otherwise indicated. During an acute stage or crisis, you may need to repeat the dosage frequently. When using homeopathy as first aid, watch the animal closely. If the remedy seems to work, but then fades out after an hour or two, repeat the remedy when its effect diminishes.

MATERIA MEDICA (ORGANIZED BY REMEDY)		

REMEDY	SYMPTOMS	DOSAGE Per day unless noted; all remedies to be given orally.
Aconitum napellus	For early stages of feverish conditions of sudden onset associated with chills, high temperature, dry skin, anxiety, intense thirst, and agitation; ailments due to fear or fright; prior to surgery	3 pellets every 1 to 2 hours (Decrease frequency with improvement.)
Allium cepa	For what appears to be a head cold or upper-respiratory infection with acrid, watery nasal discharge, mild tearing of the eyes, and sneezing; symptoms producing laryngeal discomfort; hoarseness	3 pellets every 1 to 2 hours (Decrease frequency with improvement.)
Apis mellifica	For insect stings and bites that feel better with cold applications; swollen skin or tissue that's pink or red and puffy, but when pressed, looks whitish; conditions where the tissues seem full of water (edema) (For stings and bites, remove stinger and wash well.)	3 pellets every ½ hour for 6 doses or until improvement occurs
Arnica montana	To relieve discomfort of mild trauma (accidental injuries); reduce shock and helps control bleeding; help relieve bruising; excellent after surgery	3 pellets immediately, then 3 pellets every ½ hour (Decrease frequency with improvement. Caution: Don't administer Arnica before surgery because it may interfere with anesthesia. Give it as soon as possible after surgery to help jumpstart healing.)

REMEDY	SYMPTOMS	DOSAGE Per day unless noted; all remedies to be given orally.
Arsenicum album	For gastric disturbances, diarrhea, and vomiting, or if bad food is the expected cause (Cat is anxious, restless, feels weak and cold, and frequently drinks small amounts of water.)	3 pellets 2 to 3 times a day
Belladonna	For feverish inflammatory conditions that appear suddenly and violently (Cat has a full, bounding pulse and dilation of pupils, cannot tolerate bright light, and experiences painful swallowing. Take temperature frequently. If temperature rises above 104°F [40°C],) give fluid therapy; seek veterinary care.)	3 pellets every 2 hours (Decrease frequency with improvement.)
Carbo vegetabilis	For weakness, coma, and "air hunger" where animal is having trouble breathing (Use this remedy on your way to the emergency clinic; conditions needing this remedy are extremely serious.) May also help with known carbon monoxide poisoning.	3 pellets every 10 minutes or as needed until veterinary care is obtained
Caulophyllum	For difficulties at parturition with breeding females; uterus disability, which may be accompanied by fever and thirst or tendency to retain afterbirth with accompanying bleeding; may revive labor contractions; especially helpful in establishing normal pregnancy in those who have had miscarriages	3 pellets for three to four doses
Chamomilla	For teething and accompanying gum irritation, pain, mild fever, diarrhea; for kittens who constantly whine or complain	3 pellets 3 times a day
Cocculus indicus	Mainly for motion or travel sickness with tendency to vomiting	For travel sickness: 3 pellets 1 hour before trip and then every hour, as needed (Decrease frequency with improvement.) For general malaise from travel: 3 pellets in the evening once you have arrived at your destination
Euphrasia officinalis	Mild inflammation of eyes and increased tears	3 pellets 3 to 4 times a day
Ferrum phosphoricum	Commonly used to stop bleeding (This remedy, like *Aconitum*, may be used in early stages of throat inflammations and sinus congestion.)	3 pellets 3 or 4 times a day
Hypericum perforatum	For lacerated wounds with damage to nerve endings; for injuries to the paws and toes; for spinal injuries	3 pellets every 4 hours (Decrease frequency with improvement.)
Ipecacuanha	For persistent vomiting or diarrhea usually caused by diet; may also be helpful for motion sickness	3 pellets every 15 minutes (Decrease frequency with improvement.)
Ledum palustre	To give relief from pain caused by minor puncture wounds from sharp pointed instruments such as teeth, claws, bee stings, or injections; excellent following surgery, or for insect bites and after microchipping (Affected parts are generally cold to the touch, yet feel better after cold applications.)	3 pellets every 15 minutes (Decrease frequency with improvement.)

REMEDY	SYMPTOMS	DOSAGE Per day unless noted; all remedies to be given orally.
Mercurius solubilis	For sore throat, mild fever, thirst, shivering; and excess salvation associated with a cold, thick, coated tongue; may be useful in acute stomatitis (inflammation of gums)	3 pellets every hour (Decrease frequency with improvement.)
Nux vomica	For intestinal discomfort, abdominal pain, diarrhea, indigestion, travel sickness, congestion. Helps expel hairballs and foreign bodies; also good for known ingestion of toxins	3 pellets every hour (Decrease frequency with improvement.)
Phosphorus	For dry, hard, racking cough with fever that develops rather quickly from a cold settling in the chest. Also for bleeding. (Cat craves cold food and water.)	For nosebleeds: 3 pellets immediately, repeat if needed. For other indications: 3 pellets 3 times daily
Pulsatilla	Recommended when there is a creamy, bland, thick, yellow nasal, eye, or vaginal discharge (Cat is better with cool air, cold food, and water.)	3 pellets 3 times daily (Warning: A vaginal discharge in an unspayed cat could be a uterine infection [pyometra], which is a life-threatening emergency.)
Pyrogenium	For high fevers with weak, thready pulse, or septic infections	3 pellets (200C potency) 1 time or as directed
Rhus toxicodendron	Pain and stiffness from joint conditions such as arthritis that are worse when cat first gets up but seems better after some activity. (Cold applications make symptoms worse; heat or warm compresses make them better.) Also for skin eruptions looking like poison ivy with pustules and redness	3 pellets every 6 hours
Ruta graveolens	Excellent following the use of *Arnica* for muscle soreness; also for bone pain, such as fractures or after dental extractions	3 pellets 3 times a day or until improved
Silicea	For feline acne, abscesses, and anal gland impactions. Helps expel foreign bodies such as splinters, burrs, and stingers	3 pellets 2 times a day until improved
Staphysagria	To reduce desire to spray in males after neutering	6C, 3 times daily for seven days
Symphytum officinale	Hastens healing of bone fractures; helps relieve pain and promotes healing of injured tissues, especially eyes (May be used with *Arnica*.)	3 pellets 3 to 4 times a day
Thuja occidentalis	The primary post-vaccine remedy to prevent vaccinosis; use for symptoms immediately following vaccination; also used for warts, skin tags and cysts, lipomas, and ringworm.	Dosage: 3 pellets every 12 hours for 3 doses after vaccination
Urtica urens	Helps queens to increase milk supply and later on to dry it up	To bring milk in: 3 pellets (30C) 3 times a day. To dry up milk supply: 3 pellets (6X) 3 times a day

WARNING: As with any drug, when your cat is pregnant or nursing, seek the advice of a holistic veterinarian or practitioner before using any of these remedies. When using first aid remedies, give the remedy, but don't forget to consult your vet. If symptoms persist or worsen, consult your practitioner. Keep these and all medications out of the reach of children and animals.

MINIREPERTORY (ORGANIZED BY SYMPTOM)	
SYMPTOMS	REMEDY
Abscesses	Silicea
Anal gland impactions	Silicea
Bleeding	Ferrum phosphoricum, Phosphorus
Bone fractures	Ruta graveolens, Symphytum
Bruising	Arnica montana
Deficient milk	Urtica urens (30C)
Diarrhea (dietary indiscretion)	Nux vomica, Arsenicum album
Eye injuries	Symphytum
Eyes (inflammation, tearing)	Euphrasia officinalis
Fever (sudden onset with rapid pulse)	Belladonna
High fevers, sudden infections	Belladonna
Indigestion	Nux vomica
Insect bites with swelling and redness	Apis mellifica
Motion sickness	Ipecacuana, or Cocculus indicus
Nasal discharge (bland, yellow, creamy)	Pulsatilla
Other bites or punctures	Ledum palustre
Pregnancy (stimulate uterus)	Caulophyllum
Puncture wounds, including microchips	Ledum palustre
Skin rash (sudden onset)	Arsenicum album
Sprain or strain of muscles or tendons	Arnica montana
Spraying (after neutering) or territorial behavior	Staphysagria
Surgery (post-operative only)	Arnica montana or Hypericum; for abdominal surgery use Bellis perennis
Teething	Chamomilla
Throat (sore)	Belladonna Mercurius solubilis
Trauma (general, minor)	Arnica montana
Upper respiratory symptoms with copious watery discharges	Allium cepa
Upper respiratory symptoms (early)	Aconitum napellus, Ferrum phosphoricum
Vaccinosis	Thuja
Vaginal discharge (yellow, creamy, bland)	Pulsatilla
Vomiting (nausea caused by dietary indiscretion or toxins)	Nux vomica

NOTE: Seek veterinary advice and/or consult a homeopathic practitioner prior to administration of remedies.

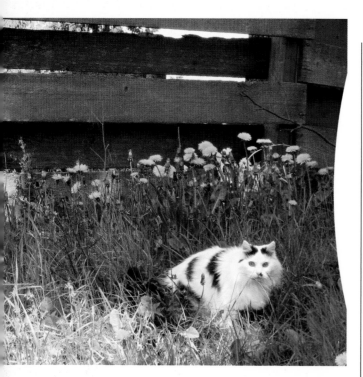

Black and White Turkish Van

FLOWER ESSENCES

Unlike antidepressants and tranquilizers, which only mask emotional distress, flower essences, or flower remedies, are gentle catalysts that alleviate underlying causes of stress and restore emotional balance. Flower remedies are benign, and they may, therefore, be safely used for humans and animals. The subtlety of this therapy makes it especially well suited to the profound emotional natures of our feline companions.

Note that flower essences are not herbal remedies. Herbs possess powerful medicinal qualities and should only be used as directed by a qualified veterinary herbalist. Flower essences do not contain any of the physical flower but only the energy or "essence" of that plant. In this way, they are somewhat like homeopathy. They're diluted to such a degree that a kind of memory or "ghost" of the original substance is imprinted on the water.

HOW TO USE FLOWER ESSENCES

Edward Bach, M.D., a British physician and flower essence inventor, reasoned that negative, inharmonious thoughts and feelings poison the system, bringing about ill health, and hindering recovery. He believed the only way to truly cure illness was to address its underlying emotional causes. This view is diametrically opposed to that of conventional medicine, which treats symptoms. Everyone—including cats—experiences negativity from time to time, but some are better able to deal with it and thus bring their systems and minds back into harmony. For those who need help, flower essences are wonderful assistants.

Flower essences are completely safe and nontoxic and do not interfere with medicines or any other healing therapies. Flower essences act on the emotions and energy and do not have direct physical effects. However, they often relieve physical symptoms whose root is emotional imbalance.

GENERAL DOSAGE INSTRUCTIONS

Giving your cat flower remedies is simple. You'll be making a dosage bottle for your combination. Choose the essences that apply to the situation; start with a maximum of six to eight remedies at a time in a combination. (Rescue Remedy counts as one essence when mixed with others.) Prepare a clean 1-ounce (30 ml) glass amber or cobalt dropper bottle by filling it with spring or purified water. Add 2 drops of each chosen remedy from its original stock bottle; for Rescue Remedy, add 4 drops. Vigorously shake the dosage bottle against your hand for a few seconds to energize the remedy. Put a few drops of the combination in the cat's food or drinking water; rub a few drops of the remedy on the inside of the cat's ears, on the crown of the head, or on the paw pads; give by mouth; and/or add a few drops to a spray bottle and spritz the environment. This works especially well for cars, carriers, and litter boxes (in the case of inappropriate elimination).

Ideally, flower remedies are given four times a day. In cases of extreme stress, Rescue Remedy may be given as often as needed. Only a few drops should be administered at a time. To increase the effect, administer essences more frequently, not in greater volume.

Administer 5 to 10 drops at a time by mouth or alternative route. Try not to touch the dropper to anything, especially the animal, so the dropper is not contaminated. If you do, rinse the dropper in hot water before you put it back into the bottle to avoid contaminating the remainder of the formula.

When the remedies are given in food or water, there's no need to worry about their effect on your other animals. If another animal (or human, for that matter) doesn't need the remedy, it will have no effect; so all your animals may freely share the same bowls. To ensure potency, always prepare the remedy-enhanced food or water fresh daily. Store flower remedies the same way you would homeopathic remedies. In other words, keep them away from sunlight, heat, strong odors, microwaves, motors, electrical equipment, and disinfecting agents.

ADDITIONAL CONSIDERATIONS: WHAT IS NORMAL?

Before you begin using flower essences, remember to look at your cats and all members of the household objectively so you know what behaviors are normal. We often accuse animals of being angry or spiteful when they behave in ways we don't like, but this is only our inability to understand animal behavior.

For example, kittens naturally bite and scratch; it is not a sign of mean-spiritedness. But since these normal behaviors aren't acceptable to us, we must find gentle ways to discourage them, or rather, to channel their normal behaviors into acceptable outlets such as toys and a scratching post.

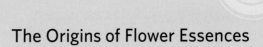

The Origins of Flower Essences

Flower essences were developed by Edward Bach, M.D. (1886–1936), an acclaimed British physician, bacteriologist, and homeopath.

After many years of researching the healing properties of flowering plants, Dr. Bach developed thirty-eight natural remedies (see "The Bach Flower Essences and Their Uses in Cats" on page 102) to alleviate every negative emotional state he identified. In addition, he created the combination formula Rescue Remedy intended for any emotionally or physically traumatic situation. Today, these remedies are world-renowned for their effectiveness.

Dr. Bach's work has had a significant influence on holistic medicine through his philosophy and essence development. However, while many of his followers believe his thirty-eight remedies are the only viable ones, other innovators have expanded the essence repertory, creating thousands of new essences of not only other flowers but animals and even inanimate objects (gems, crystals, minerals, mountains, lakes, landmarks) and the intangible (celestial bodies and even angelic beings).

THE BACH FLOWER ESSENCES AND THEIR USES IN CATS

Dr. Bach's thirty-eight flower essences comprise a simple system that is easy to use at home for your cat and other family members. Just select the remedies that seem most applicable to the situation you are treating. For instance, if you have two cats that are jealous of each other and fight, look for remedies that address jealousy, anger, communication, and the need for attention. Use your intuition to create new combinations of flower remedies suitable for your cats.

AGRIMONY (*Agrimonia eupatoria*): This flower essence is used for animals that have difficulty communicating; symptoms due to repressed emotions; skin irritations; feral cats that cannot adjust to captivity; and nocturnal restlessness.

ASPEN (*Populus tremula*): For the "scaredy-cat" that slinks from one safe place to another and startles easily at any sound, even nonthreatening ones. Aspen promotes groundedness and a sense of security in the home. Aspen is for general, nonspecific fears while Mimulus is the correct remedy for known or specific fears. The root of fear in the Aspen personality is a lack of connection with other animals or humans, (shown at left).

BEECH (*Fagus sylvatica*): For cats who are intolerant of other animals, certain people, or even certain situations, Beech is appropriate. It can be helpful for the cat that sprays on the belongings of his owner's new mate. Also, Beech can alleviate general irritation. It's also helpful for picky eaters to tolerate dietary changes. Combine it with Walnut for keeping peace between cats that always fight.

CENTAURY (*Centaurium erythaea*): This essence is appropriate for the quiet, submissive cat or the cat that allows himself to be bullied or abused by a dog, a child, or another cat. Centaury increases the will to live when fighting an illness or during a challenging labor and delivery.

CERATO (*Ceratostigma willmottiana*): This essence is for flighty, inattentive animals; it is valuable during shows or training sessions, when a cat's ability to focus is required. It's also excellent for anxiety and related problems, such as feline eating disorders, especially during pregnancy.

CHERRY PLUM (*Prunus cerasifera*): This is one of the ingredients in Rescue Remedy. It's useful for the cat that loses self-control and becomes wild and vicious when stressed by strange people, the smell of other animals, or unfamiliar noises. It's also used for retaining control during heat cycles and/or mating (for both sexes). It's good for pregnant queens that seem unusually stressed and for the cat that constantly chews himself or chases his own tail. It may be helpful in case of seizures, incontinence, and allergies, and to help cats stop biting at sutures after surgery.

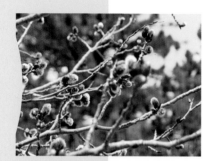

Aspen (*Populus tremula*)

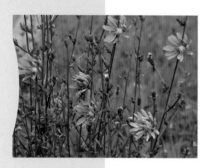

Chicory (*Cichorium intybus*)

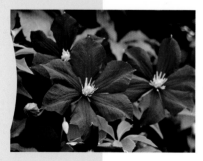

Clematis (*Clematis vitalba*)

CHESTNUT BUD (*Ceratostigma willmottiana*): This essence is used to break bad habits or during training sessions to increase memory retention and a keen sense of awareness. It helps cats learn lessons necessary for coexisting peacefully in a human environment such as not to scratch the couch.

CHICORY (*Cichorium intybus*): Use this flower essence for the clingy cat, which may be possessive, manipulative, and jealous (wanting always to be near you, to be held, petted, and fussed over); for the mother cat that is overly possessive with her litter, especially when it's time for her kittens to leave home; and for the cat that thinks she owns the house or seeks attention in negative ways, (shown opposite, left).

CLEMATIS (*Clematis vitalba*): This is one of the ingredients in Rescue Remedy. When the cat appears stunned or experiences unusual, prolonged patterns of sleep beyond the typical catnap, try this essence. It's also used to help regain consciousness following surgery or injury, (shown opposite, left).

CRAB APPLE (*Malus sylvestris*): This remedy is especially cleansing during or after any illness, rash, open wound, or parasite infestation. It's used to detoxify and heal. It also helps cats with poor self-image that cower during shows, or cats previously abused or abandoned.

ELM (*Ulmus procera*): Consider this flower essence for the cat that becomes overwhelmed when he must change location, go to the groomer, or be subjected to too many people at a time, such as a cat show or when visitors come to the home, (shown at right).

GENTIAN (*Gentiana amerella*): Give this essence for setbacks of any kind, such as when the cat gets worse before he gets better during the course of an illness, arthritis symptoms, or rehabilitation from surgery. It helps to give cats inner fortitude to deal with whatever comes their way and instills optimism, (shown at right).

GORSE (*Ulex europaeus*): This essence may be used for apathy, depression, and despair, when the cat refuses to eat or to improve, or when battling cancer, a critical injury, major surgery, or long-term illness.

HEATHER (*Calluna vulgaris*): For the center-of-attention cat that cries for attention or when left alone. For the cat being boarded or housed in a shelter, consider this essence, (shown at right).

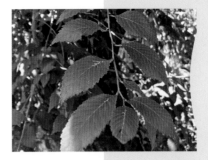

Elm (*Ulmus procera*)

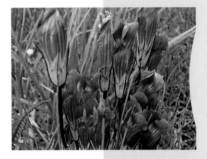

Gentian (*Gentiana amerella*)

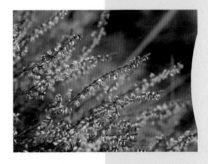

Heather (*Calluna vulgaris*)

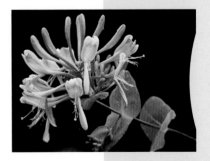

Honeysuckle (*Lonicera caprifolium*)

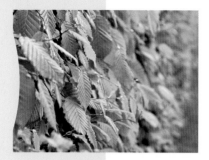

Hornbeam (*Carpinus betulus*)

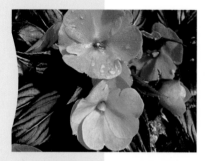

Impatiens (*Impatiens gladulifera*)

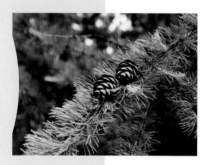

Larch (*Larix deciua*)

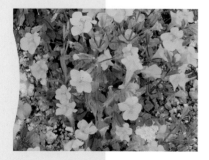

Mimulus (*Mimulus guttatus*)

HOLLY (*Ilex aquifolium*): For the angry or jealous cat with a hair-trigger temper, for cats who are unable to receive love and affection, and especially good for abused or neglected cats that may need to be quarantined, rescued cats, and feral cats. This essence helps to nourish the heart and release jealousy, rage, and anger.

HONEYSUCKLE (*Lonicera caprifolium*): This flower essence helps cats stop grieving after change such as a new home or loss of loved one, whether by death or separation. It may help after a long birthing experience, for the mother caring for her young after a cesarean section, or to help the cat release the past and adjust to new situations, (shown page 103).

HORNBEAM (*Carpinus betulus*): For fatigue and lack of vitality, this strengthening remedy is helpful in assisting the runt of the litter or building up any sickly animal, (shown at left).

IMPATIENS (*Impatiens gladulifera*): This flower essence is one of the ingredients in Rescue Remedy. Consider it for the cat that gets agitated by too much excitement or that is overly anxious at mealtimes or before a cat show. It promotes patience, tolerance, and acceptance, and it's also good for pain, (shown at left).

LARCH (*Larix deciua*): For a cat low in the cat hierarchy of the household, or the runt of the litter, this remedy may help. For the cat with low self-esteem it increases self-confidence; especially helpful before a cat show or event so he can hold his head high, (shown at left).

MIMULUS (*Mimulus guttatus*): This essence is for fear of specific things or circumstances—such as thunderstorms, dogs, doorbells, vacuums, car rides, and children. It's also useful for deep fears, such as fear of starving, strangers, and abandonment. When fear turns to terror, use Rock Rose or Rescue Remedy. It is helpful for illnesses that don't respond to treatment, such as post influenza, (shown at left).

MUSTARD (*Sinapis arvensis*): Try this flower essence for the depressed cat, especially if complicated by hormonal changes such as a kitten coming into heat for the first time, the stud discovering girls, during pregnancy if depression is noticeable, or if the cat is cantankerous during heat. It promotes serenity and optimism, especially in older cats, (shown at right).

OAK (*Quercus robur*): For physical exhaustion, such as the last weeks of pregnancy, when the cat feels overburdened, for long chronic illness, or to rebuild strength after harsh living conditions, starvation, or abuse, (shown at right).

OLIVE (*Olea europaea*): This essence is beneficial for mental and emotional exhaustion following a long ordeal or long-term pain, for elderly cats that become exhausted easily, for the cat plagued by stressed adrenals or allergies, and for caged cats that exhaust themselves trying to get out, (shown at right).

PINE (*Pinus sylvestris*): For the cat given away or left behind, this flower essence clears guilt and shame. In competition, this is for the cat that never makes it to the finals though she's show quality. For the cat that looks guilty whenever her human companion is upset, even though it isn't the cat's fault, (shown at right).

RED CHESTNUT (*Aesculus carnea*): This remedy helps alleviate overconcern for others: the cat that constantly watches out the window when his human companion is late coming home, or the mother worrying over her kittens. It's also helpful for separation anxiety.

RESCUE REMEDY (a combination of Star of Bethlehem, Rock Rose, Impatiens, Clematis, and Cherry Plum): Try this classic for any kind of trauma. In the case of an accident, see your veterinarian immediately. However, Rescue Remedy can help you through the trauma of getting the cat to the veterinarian's office. It's used on pregnant queens, on car trips, for boarding, during long absences from home, before and after surgery, or whenever the cat experiences unusual stress. Also, it can stop a seizure very quickly. Rescue Remedy helps newborn kittens wake up and breathe. Give them one drop every few minutes on the tips of the ears or on the paw pads.

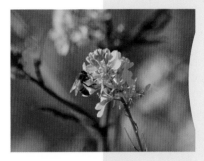

Mustard (*Sinapis arvensis*)

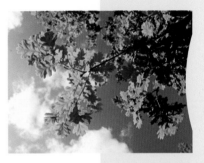

Oak (*Quercus robur*)

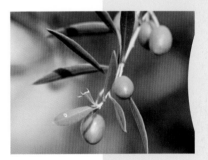

Olive (*Olea europaea*)

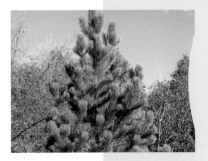

Pine (*Pinus sylvestris*)

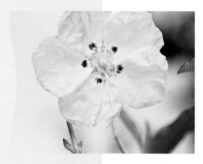

Rock Rose
(Helianthemum nummularium)

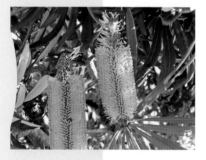

Star of Bethlehem
(Ornithogalum umbellatum)

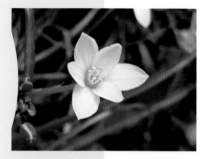

Vervain (*Verbena officinalis*)

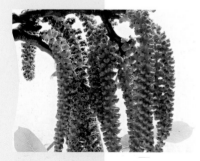

Walnut (*Juglans regia*)

ROCK ROSE (*Helianthemum nummularium*): This is one of the ingredients in Rescue Remedy. Use it immediately for cats that experience panic or terror, especially after an accident, injury, or other terrifying event, (shown at left).

ROCK WATER (solarized spring water): For stiffness and rigidity of mind or body, this essence promotes increased joint flexibility and mental resiliency. It's helpful for picky, inflexible eaters.

SCLERANTHUS (*Scleranthus annuus*): This flower essence promotes balance and stability. It can be used for the cat with equilibrium problems or neurological confusion, as in some kinds of seizures, deafness, dizziness, head tilt, inner ear infection, or vestibular disease, or complications to one side (such as stroke or partial paralysis).

STAR OF BETHLEHEM (*Ornithogalum umbellatum*): This is one of the ingredients in Rescue Remedy. Consider it for all trauma—physical, mental, and emotional, such as loss of loved one, injury, abuse, and birthing difficulties. Use it to comfort cats boarded in a kennel or hospitalized for any reason, (shown at left).

SWEET CHESTNUT (*Castanea sativa*): For the high-strung cat at its wit's end, for the cat forced to remain in a kennel or carrier for long periods (for instance, to recover from orthopedic surgery), to prevent burnout in show cats, or any time the cat needs extra endurance or energy, give this essence a try.

VERVAIN (*Verbena officinalis*): Use this essence for the intense, hyperactive, or very high-strung cat; combine it with Vine for "bullies," (shown at left).

VINE (*Vitis vinifera*): Vine helps relax the dominant "top cat" who thinks he's in charge or the strong-willed cat who rules with claws rather than velvet paws.

WALNUT (*Juglans regia*): This flower essence is helpful for any type of change or transition, including weaning and heat cycles. It eases adjustment to houseguests, holidays, a new home, changes in schedule, roommates moving in or out, new diet, etc. It is also helpful for the very sensitive cat who is easily disturbed, (shown at left).

WATER VIOLET (*Hottonia palustris*): This is a constitutional remedy for most cats. It helps them keep their instinct for solitude in balance with the enjoyment of interactions with people and other animals in their environment. It's also used for grief, loneliness, and lack of joy, (shown at right).

WHITE CHESTNUT (*Aesculus hippocastanum*): This essence is used for repetitive thoughts and behaviors, as well as for that cat who worries about her grown kittens, (shown at right).

WILD OATS (*Bromus ramosus*): This essence can be used for the bored cat that doesn't feel useful anymore, such as the retired show cat, for the cat that chews curtains or furniture out of boredom, and in competitions, where the cat needs to have a strong desire to win, (shown at right).

WILD ROSE (*Rosa canina*): This flower essence is useful for cats to remain content under any circumstances, for older cats when you bring a new kitten home, for the older, grouchy cat, or the cat placed in a cage during a cat show, (shown at right).

WILLOW (*Salix vitellina*): Use this essence for situations of resentment, such as the cat that ignores you when you come home because you left it alone all day or the retired show cat that misses that attention. It promotes acceptance and forgiveness.

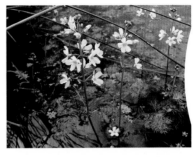

Water Violet (*Hottonia palustris*)

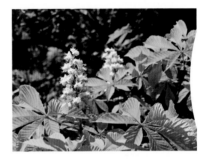

White Chestnut (*Aesculus hippocastanum*)

FLOWER REMEDY COMBINATIONS

Flower remedies work very well in combination. Many wonderful multi-essence blends are available that are designed for specific behaviors and situations (see Flower Essences under Suppliers on page 175). Or, use your intuition to fashion Bach flower mixtures that are right for your cat. Here are a few ideas.

EMOTIONAL HEALING FORMULA (for stray, shelter, abused, or neglected cats): Aspen, Larch, Star of Bethlehem

TRAVEL/TRANSITION FORMULA: Rescue Remedy, Elm, Walnut, Mimulus, Scleranthus

HEALING AND RECOVERY FORMULA: Crab Apple, Gentian, Gorse, Walnut, Sweet Chestnut, Olive, Honeysuckle

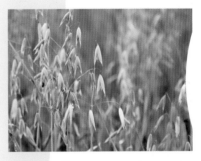

Wild Oats (*Bromus ramosus*)

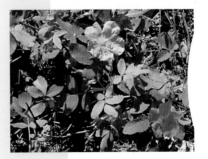

Wild Rose (*Rosa canina*)

Avoid Synthetic Scents

Just like synthetic vitamins, synthetic oils are missing life energy and so should never be used in veterinary aromatherapy. A true essential oil comes from living things, and thus has a direct link with the Earth, a subtle energy that can't be duplicated in a laboratory. The energies of these plant materials merge with our own and those of our cats to support healing. For example, genuine rose oil envelops us in scent and guides us through a field of flowers. A synthetic rose oil is more likely to give you a headache and repel your cat.

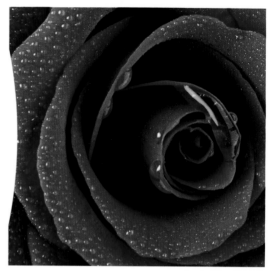

Red rose (*rosea rubra*)

AROMATHERAPY

The subtle, careful use of aromatherapy can enhance all healing therapies, especially for cats, whose sense of smell is so much more complex and acute than our own. The olfactory ability is the result of evolution: The acuteness of cats' senses allowed them to evade predators and other dangers in the wilderness.

Humans use aromatherapy to stimulate the immune system and promote healing, typically employing essential oils—the distilled or expressed product of aromatic plant materials. Aromatic essences have many desirable qualities: They may be antibacterial, antiviral, antispasmodic, and diuretic; some are vasodilators or vasoconstrictors (widening or narrowing blood vessels, respectively); and others act on the adrenals, ovaries, and thyroid glands.

Aromatherapy must always be used safely and appropriately. *Never* apply an essential oil directly to the cat's skin or fur. Many oils are toxic and will be absorbed through the skin, which can make the cat extremely ill. Before using aromatherapy with your cat, allow her to smell a drop of the oil which has been rubbed between your palms to make sure it isn't aversive. All essential oils must be diluted at least 1:10 in a carrier oil (such as olive or almond oil); even better, buy essential oils in the hydrosol form (water extract). Always provide an escape route for the cat, so that she can get away if she does not like the smell or it becomes too overwhelming.

Hydrosols are convenient sprays that can be misted around the cat's bedding and toys and may also be sprayed into a room just like an air freshener. In zoo environments, many keepers will use a few drops of a fragrance such as vanilla (*Vanilla planifolia*) extract (we recommend organic) on a piece of cotton cloth and let the exotic cats investigate the scent. You can try this with the cat's fabric toys instead of sprinkling them with or stuffing them with catnip (*Nepeta cataria*). There are also catnip hydrosols, which many cats find fascinating.

When showing cats, a whiff of bay rum or organic vanilla extract applied to a cotton pad prior to a show ring appearance is helpful to distract from the scent of other cats.

Common basil (*Ocimum basilicum*), calendula (*Calendula officinalis*), Roman chamomile (*Anthemis nobilis*), rosemary (*Rosmarinus officinalis*), and valerian (*Valeriana officinalis*) are also scents that seem to attract cats. Try the following hydrosols, singly or in combination, to assist in a variety of circumstances.

FOR CALMING: lavender (*Lavandula* spp.), rose (*Rosa damascena*), scented geranium (*Pelargonium graveolens*), neroli (*Citrus aurantium var. amara* or *Bigaradia* blossom)

FOR COMFORT: calendula (*Calendula officinalis*)

FOR COURAGE: sweet pea (*Lathyrus odoratus*), yarrow (*Achillea millefolium*)

FOR DEPRESSION: jasmine (*Jasminum grandiflorum*)

FOR HEALING: coriander (*Coriandrum sativum*), cypress (*Cupressus sempervirens*), myrrh (*Commiphora myrrha*), lavender (*Lavandula* spp.), palmarosa (rose geranium) (*Cymbopogon martini*)

FOR LONGEVITY: sweet fennel (*Foenicum vulgare*), rosemary (*Rosmarinus officinalis*)

FOR SLEEP AND CALMING: chamomile (*Anthemis nobilis*), hyacinth (*Hyacinthus orientalis*), jasmine (*Jasminum grandiflorum*), lavender (*Lavandula* spp.)

TO CLEAN WOUNDS OR BURNS: lavender (*Lavandula* spp.), rose (*Rosa damascena*), geranium (*Pelargonium graveolens*), chamomile (*Anthemis nobilis*)

ESSENTIAL OIL PRECAUTIONS

Keep essential oils and hydrosols away from strong light, heat, air, and moisture. Never let any living being lick, eat, or drink them; never add them to food or water. Watch for allergic reactions, and be sure that animals and children don't have direct access to the oils.

The following essential oils are toxic or aversive to cats. Note: All citrus oils made from fruit peels are aversive to cats.

- Bergamot (bitter orange) (*Citrus aurantium spp. bergamia*)
- Birch (*Betula* spp.)
- Cinnamon (*Cinnamomum zeylanicum*)
- Clove (*Syzygium aromaticum*)
- Fir (*Abies* spp.)
- Grapefruit (*Citrus paradisi*)
- Lemon (*Citrus limonum*)
- Lime (*Citrus aurantifolia*)
- Mandarin Orange (*Citrus reticulata*)
- Niaouli (*Melaleuca quinquenervia*)
- Orange (sweet) (*Citrus sinensis*)
- Oregano (*Origanum vulgare*)
- Pine (*Pinus* spp.)
- Sage (*Salvia officinalis*)
- Savory (*Satureja hortensis*)
- Spruce (*Picea* spp.)
- Tangerine (*Citrus reticulata*)
- Tea Tree (*Melaleuca alternifolia*)
- Thyme (*Thymus vulgaris*)

6

HANDS-ON HEALING

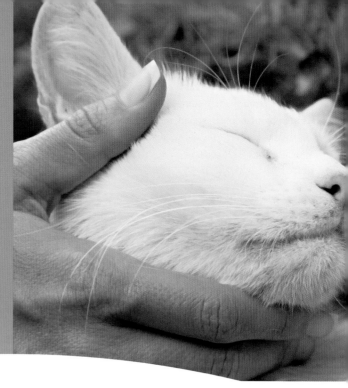

Most cats readily accept a healing touch.

Many hands-on therapeutic interventions normally associated with human healing are also beneficial to cats. Some involve direct physical intervention, and others are more energetic in nature, but all of them seek to realign and restore the body's correct function. When everything is properly aligned and qi (chi) is flowing without hindrances or blockages, the body is able to dispose of toxins, clear out inflammation, reduce stress, and prevent new problems—and thus reduce the ravaging effects of aging.

Regardless of what modalities you choose, if you approach your cat with honor and respect, the therapy will most likely be welcome. Consult your holistic veterinarian before embarking on any course of treatment. (For sources of further information about many of the treatments described here, see Resources on page 174.)

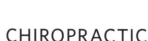

CHIROPRACTIC

Chiropractic, a method of manipulating bones and joints, is one of the most popular and widely used holistic therapies. Applying chiropractic to cats is not such a strange idea, since they have many of the same musculoskeletal problems that people do. Many veterinarians are certified in chiropractic techniques and can work effectively to restore healthy function to your cat.

The basic principle of chiropractic is to correct *subluxations*, which are small misalignments between vertebrae that may not even be visible on x-rays. (A luxation is a complete dislocation.) A subluxation affects peripheral nerves at the root level, where the nerves exit between the vertebrae. It puts pressure on the sensitive nerve root, thus interfering with its function. This pinched nerve is usually painful, and it may also cause functional problems in the organs fed by that nerve. Surrounding muscles may go into spasm, which is also painful and restricts movement. The chiropractor realigns the vertebrae by applying gentle force to specific points along the spine, thus reducing pain and inflammation.

Cats have a reputation for grace, but they can still do clumsy things. They may land wrong when jumping or bump into furniture while playing. These physical jolts can push the spine out of alignment. If your cat becomes touchy or grumpy, it may not be her attitude that needs adjusting—she may be trying to communicate pain.

Laws may restrict or prohibit chiropractors from working on animals, so consult your veterinarian before seeking chiropractic treatment for your cat. It's best to find a practitioner who is certified and trained in adjusting small animals. An unqualified practitioner may inadvertently do great harm to the delicate feline skeletal system. A thrust at the wrong angle could injure the cat permanently.

Because spinal misalignments often involve muscle spasms, or even scarring in the case of long-standing problems, a series of adjustments may be needed to retrain the muscles and joints to stay in their natural position. Periodic "tune-ups" are also helpful in preventing minor problems from becoming deeply established.

NETWORK SPINAL ANALYSIS

A particular type of chiropractic, Network Spinal Analysis, was created by chiropractor Donald Epstein, D.C. This technique involves gentle, precise touch to the spine. It promotes spontaneous release of spinal and life tensions, and it uses existing tension as fuel for spinal reorganization and enhanced wellness. Dr. Epstein theorizes that most spinal problems originate in tension along the whole spinal system due to physical, mental, and/or emotional traumas from which the animal has not been able to recover fully. These effects are additive if not addressed and released, and eventually they may result in dysfunction and pain. This pain may originate from physical trauma, or it may be the result of ongoing tensions that build up until symptoms become overt. Network Spinal Analysis is extremely gentle and works very well for cats.

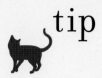

tip

Uses of Chiropractic

Chiropractic medicine may also be used to treat certain internal disorders. It is most helpful when an internal disorder has just begun. In very advanced cases, it may not be as effective, though it can certainly be an important stepping stone toward healing.

Chiropractic isn't the correct treatment for fractures, infectious diseases, abscesses, or blocked urinary tracts. It's best to have a veterinarian examine the cat before employing chiropractic therapy. Radiographs (x-rays) are needed to determine whether a fracture is present or if there is another reason the cat should not be adjusted by a chiropractor.

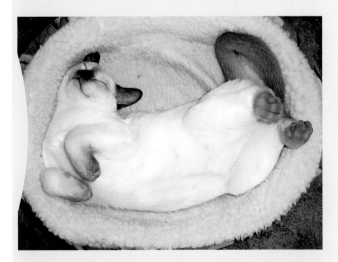

Cat Fanciers' Association's Premier Celestecats Matrix, Champagne Point Tonkinese, sixth generation raw food-fed cat

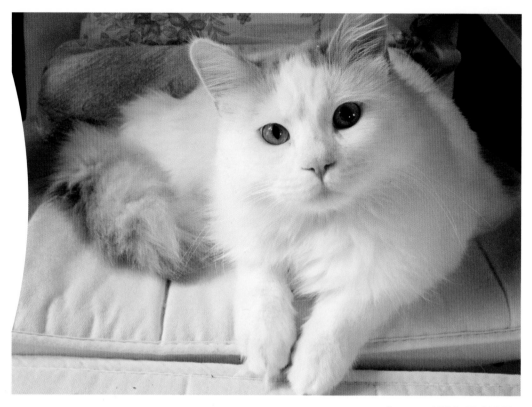

Cream and White Turkish Van

VETERINARY ORTHOPEDIC MANIPULATION

Veterinary orthopedic manipulation (VOM) is a healing technology that locates areas of the animal's nervous system that have fallen out of communication with each other. Every cell in the body communicates with other cells as well as with all body systems. VOM helps re-establish neuronal communication and thus induces healing. VOM is a simple, effective, and safe healing modality. It is an objective, fast, and easy-to-apply technology that takes a minimum of time to master. VOM is different from chiropractic care; it has similarities to some of the chiropractic modalities and functions in restoring function by reducing subluxations. VOM delivers its force with a hand-held device called a *spinal accelerometer*, which is similar to the activator that is commonly used by chiropractors. It looks a bit like a spring-loaded doorstop.

ACUPUNCTURE

Acupuncture, a technique that stimulates specific points in the body to rectify energetic imbalances, originated more than 2,000 years ago in China. According to one legend, someone noticed that lame war horses, when wounded by arrows in certain spots, would stop limping. (Another legend tells a similar tale about humans.) The same spots were stimulated in other lame horses, and they also stopped limping.

Human and veterinary acupuncture had unique origins, using different charts. The human charts showed a system of interconnected pathways (meridians and collaterals) through which the body's energy flows. Hundreds of acupuncture points are spread throughout these pathways.

After the meridians of the body were discovered and mapped, it was concluded that any disruption of the energy flow, qi (chi), caused disease. The placement of small needles along exact points on these meridians was found to enhance the flow of qi and promote a state of health.

Originally, stone needles were used. Today acupuncturists choose from metal needles, heat, pressure, massage, electrical stimulation, injections, magnets, gold beads, lasers, or any combination of these methods to stimulate a point.

Identification of animal meridians was done independently, and their points were usually given different names from human ones, even when the location and function seemed identical. Charts were developed primarily for farm animals, especially the horse, chicken, pig, and water buffalo. Today in China, though cats and dogs are treated with acupuncture, the emphasis is still on farm animals.

In the United States, acupuncture has been considered a valid method of treatment by the American Veterinary Medical Association for decades. Many holistic veterinarians embrace this technique in their practices. To become a certified veterinary acupuncturist, a practitioner must complete a year-long training course and pass a certification examination.

Although acupuncture, like many treatments in western medicine, may be used to treat symptoms alone, the best approach is to correct the underlying imbalances that created the conditions fostering specific diseases. Most contemporary acupuncturists emphasize a total approach to health and include in their practice advice on the use of clinical nutrition, herbs, and the like.

PREPARING FOR AN ACUPUNCTURE TREATMENT

As with homeopathy, it's important to glean as much information about the cat's general habits, attitude, background, and family life before the treatment. Placement of the needles may be determined by such factors as the personality and characteristics of the cat, the time of day the problem occurs, and the kind of weather that makes it worse.

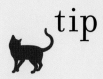

tip

An Ancient Technique for Modern Cats

Animal acupuncture is used to treat many conditions such as arthritis, spinal and disc problems, kidney disorders, metabolic imbalances, aging disorders, cataracts, asthma, and allergic dermatitis.

Acupuncture has also been used as an anesthetic; studies have shown that endorphins and encephalins (pain relievers produced naturally by the body) are released when certain acupuncture points are stimulated.

During the physical exam, the anatomy of the cat is examined, as are acupuncture points along the spine. A specific point may be tender or painful when a cat has a problem with organs or meridians associated with that point. Some veterinary acupuncturists also use conventional tests such as blood panels, radiographs, and stool tests to help them assess the animal's condition.

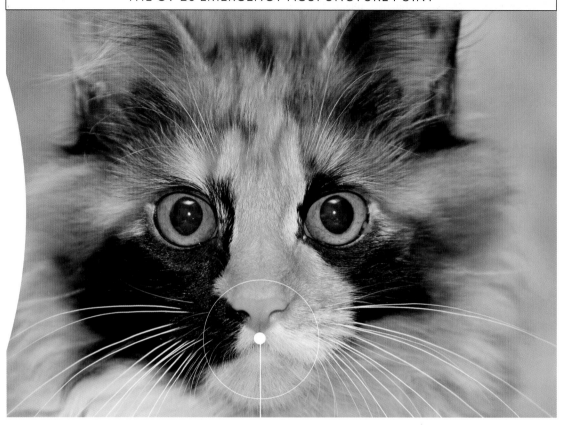

GV-26 is the emergency or resuscitation point. You can stimulate it with a pin, pen point, or even a fingernail. Nonbreathing newborns or sick or traumatized cats can sometimes be resuscitated this way.

THE EFFECTS OF ACUPUNCTURE

One acupuncture treatment usually offers relief, but multiple treatments are usually required before dramatic and lasting results are seen. The most difficult thing about acupuncture, as with homeopathy, is that some cats may get worse before they get better. But once through the crisis, their improvement may be dramatic and enduring.

You may wonder how your cat will tolerate acupuncture. Many holistic veterinarians report that cats who resist treatment at the first session often prove extremely cooperative in subsequent visits. Many times the cat will let the practitioner know where it hurts, and then purr throughout the treatment. The most difficult part about an acupuncture treatment is practical: Many cats will not sit still for the ten minutes needed. Acupuncturists may use a variation called aquapuncture, in which they inject small quantities of liquid, such as a solution of vitamin B12 and lidocaine, or homeopathic or other remedies, at the therapeutic points. Acupuncture points can also be treated with finger pressure, lasers, and other techniques.

Cats who have long suffered with chronic disease, such as arthritis, often enjoy relief through acupuncture, especially if nutrition and other holistic treatments are included in the healing regimen. Since acupuncture is very good for reducing inflammation, as well as improving energy and information flow throughout the body's nervous and immune systems, it is an excellent antiaging therapy for cats.

Note that acupuncture may interfere with homeopathy, and the two therapies aren't often used together. If your cat is being treated with classical homeopathy, ask your practitioner if she advises using both therapies simultaneously.

THERAPEUTIC TOUCH

Therapeutic touch (TTouch) therapy, a method devised by Linda Tellington-Jones, is a type of nonverbal communication through cellular memory. The practitioner speaks to the cellular intelligence in her hands, which in turn speaks to the cells in the body. When working on animals, simply by placing your hands on the body and moving them in a circular manner, you create a kind of kinesthetic (sensory) interspecies communication.

Tellington-Jones initially studied the Feldenkreis Method, which opens new neurological pathways to the brain through the use of nonhabitual movements. She then developed her own techniques based on Feldenkreis's work, beginning with the concept that every cell in the body knows its function. The use of the circular movement, when done with respect, increases the speed of healing at the cellular level.

Animals may actually be born with "habitual holding patterns," but even the most resistant animals respond to this technique and learn to release stuck energy.

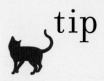

A Simple Technique to Get You Started

Here's a very simple technique that many touch therapists recommend. Hold your hands, if your cat will allow it, over a painful spot. See if you can let positive healing energy flow from you via your right hand into your cat, and let any negative or painful energy flow from the cat into your left hand. (If you are more comfortable using the opposite hand, this is fine, too.) Afterward—and this is very important for your self-care as a healer—shake your hands to release any negative energy from your body. Let the cat rest comfortably and use this healing energy in her own way.

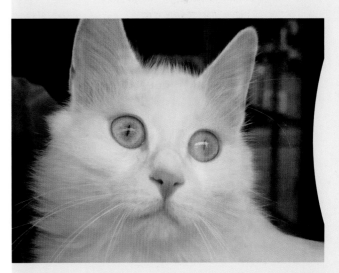

Odd-eyed White Turkish Van

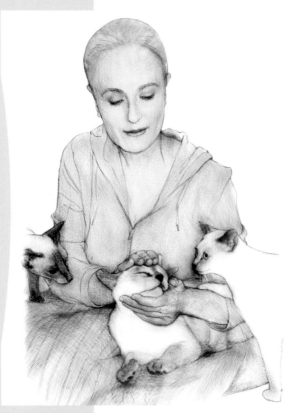

Practicing TTouch on Romeo

HOW TO PRACTICE TTOUCH

TTouch involves making little circles all over the cat's body (or just where needed). Imagine the face of a small clock, 1 to 2 inches (2.5 to 5 cm) in diameter, where you touch your cat. Begin at six o'clock and gently push the skin clockwise all the way around, past six and finish at nine. At nine o'clock, pause, lift your fingers, and begin again in another spot. It's important to maintain a constant pressure and close the circles. Use your middle three fingers and make 1¼ circles at each spot, then move on and repeat. Rest your thumb and fourth finger (pinkie) against the cat's body to steady your hand. This circular touch is called the *clouded leopard touch*.

Do not repeat the same spot twice and don't connect three circles in a row (which we all tend to do initially). Remember to lift your fingers as you close each circle and begin again. You may also use your left hand. (Generally, you would use your dominant hand, but for a larger animal, such as a big dog or horse, you may use both hands.)

Allow your hands to find their own way as they communicate with the cells of your animal companion. Try to tune into her breathing and her response to your touch. You may find your own breathing falls into sync with your cat's. Concentrate on making the circles and on sensing the animal's response. And, as always, approach your cat with respect.

THE BENEFITS OF TTOUCH

The circular motion (and other techniques) of TTouch seems to imprint on the animal's cells more than simple petting or stroking, which although loving and beneficial, doesn't seem to activate the cellular awareness in the same way. In addition to improving lymphatic and blood flow, TTouch is an excellent way to reduce stress in cats, which may even provide life-extension and antiaging benefits. (See "Hands-On Healing" in Resources on page 174 for sources of additional information on learning this technique.)

REIKI: UNIVERSAL LIFE FORCE ENERGY

Profound healing is possible through the power of touch. The Reiki practitioner, an initiated individual, channels energy in the form of pure white light to heal. Reiki originated in Tibet thousands of years ago, and its history may be traced through India, Egypt, Ephesus, Greece, Rome, China, and Japan, and from there to the West.

Reiki is not dependent on the energy clarity or healing ability of the practitioner. In other healing modalities, the conscious and subconscious belief system of the energy practitioner may affect the outcome of their chosen healing modality. With Reiki, the practitioner only serves as a conduit for the flow of pure white healing light; thus no negative energy is absorbed by or sent between the healer and the patient.

Reiki differs from other hands on-healing modalities by requiring a series of four *attunements*, which are like energetic initiations. These attunements activate and set the energy path in the practitioner. This energy path remains active for the practitioner's entire life. It runs through the chakra system and ultimately to the hands. Whenever an initiated individual touches anything with the intention to help or heal, the Reiki energy automatically flows through their hands with no effort or expenditure on the practitioner's part.

REIKI ATTUNEMENTS

To give an attunement, the practitioner must be a Reiki master. The First Degree Reiki attunement activates the healing energy so that it flows when anything is physically touched with intention. The Second Degree Reiki attunement activates the energy so that it flows when certain symbols are performed by the Reiki practitioner, who can then activate healing at any distance, even without physically being present. The Third Degree or Master Reiki attunement activates the healing energy that sets the Reiki pathways in another individual.

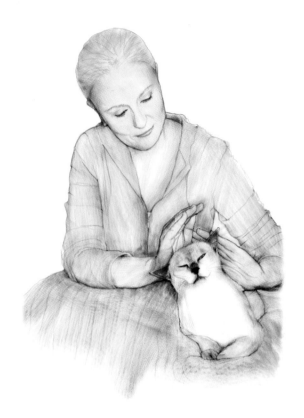

Doing Reiki on Juliette

THE BENEFITS OF REIKI

The Reiki method of healing may be used on plants, animals, and people from infants to the elderly. It has been effective in treating everything from mild imbalances to life-threatening illnesses. Reiki is a wonderful antiaging technique because it increases blood flow to areas where it was restricted, thereby allowing the body to cleanse itself more deeply. Reiki can also realign muscles, nerves, and even bones, improving energy and information flow throughout the body.

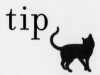

tip

Celeste's Special Massage

My cats and kittens love this massage. If your cat does not mind lying on her back on your lap, place her between your thighs, with your knees together, with the cat's head resting on your knees and the hind feet toward your tummy. Hold your cat with your thumbs under her armpits, and all of your fingers (both hands) on the cat's neck. Commence a deep kneading action with your fingers and nails (if short enough) into her neck. Work from behind the ears, down into the shoulders. When done correctly, your cat will relax into utter bliss. Don't worry if she tolerates this only briefly and then scoots away at first; she'll most likely come to love it. This is an excellent way to end a massage session.

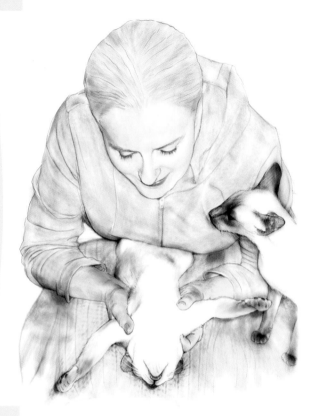

Celeste's special massage on Juliette

Within the Reiki community of practitioners, many specialize in working with animals. The animal Reiki practitioner often receives intuitive information from the animal during treatment. This information is helpful to the animal's human companion in understanding what their animal friend is going through at the time. Cats are especially good at living in the moment, and they appreciate as much stress reduction as possible for not only themselves but their human companions as well.

The Reiki animal practitioner can be an extremely valuable ally to your doctor of veterinary medicine. However, since there is so little known about energy medicine and its healing modalities in western veterinary medicine, it can often become difficult to include a Reiki practitioner in your cat's therapy. If you find a holistic veterinarian who is a Reiki practitioner, you are indeed fortunate.

MASSAGE THERAPY

Most cats love to be petted, and massage seems to feel even better. Start with the paws, legs, abdomen, torso, spine, and neck, head, and ears.

No special training is required to perform massage, although it's helpful to learn a number of specific movements. When you're petting your cat, just go a little deeper and gently knead and move the muscles under the skin. Cats seem to especially enjoy a good neck massage.

When pregnant queens are in labor, a light, gentle circular massage on their bellies (called *effleurage* in Lamaze natural childbirth classes for people) is a gentle massage technique much appreciated by cat mothers-to-be. Effleurage helps reduce stress and makes for a very pleasant birthing experience.

THE NAMBUDRIPAD ALLERGY ELIMINATION TECHNIQUE

The Nambudripad Allergy Elimination Technique (NAET) is a diagnostic and treatment technique based on the principles of Chinese Medicine and acupuncture. It was developed for humans by Devi Nambudripad D.C., L.Ac., R.N., Ph.D. Veterinarians have extended the use of NAET to domestic pets. NAET can be performed in the vet's office or over the phone. Factors that contribute to premature aging, such as emotional trauma and other stressors, can be offset with use of NAET because it is so effective at calming the immune system and reducing inflammation.

Allergies are one of the most common problems that pets face today. While, strictly speaking, an allergy is a very specific type of immune reaction, usually to a protein, in NAET, allergies are considered to be an unusual sensitivity to any substance. Allergies may result from repeated exposure to an allergen over a long period of time (food allergies are a common example), brief exposure to a very strong or toxic substance, or from events such as serious trauma, major surgery, and vaccination.

NAET offers an energy-medicine solution to allergic conditions. Muscle testing (see "Applied Kinesiology" on page 134) is used to confirm the presence of allergic reactivity. Once identified, acupuncture and/or acupressure is used to eliminate the allergy by reprogramming the body's response to future contact. A specific protocol has been developed that prioritizes treatment of common as well as unique allergens. (NAET training is only available to professionals. See the Resources, page 174, to find a practitioner.)

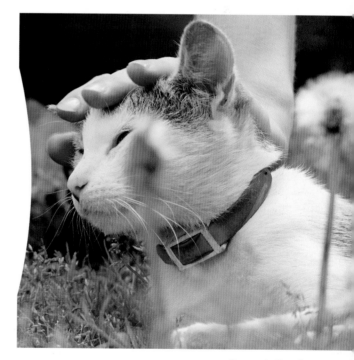

Domestic Shorthair

EMOTIONAL FREEDOM TECHNIQUES

Emotional Freedom Techniques (EFT) is a method of tapping certain points along traditional Chinese acupuncture meridians in order to resolve emotional, behavioral, and physical problems. EFT, one of the new school of meridian energy therapies, was developed by Gary Craig. By tapping on these points while keeping a specific problem in mind, negative energy is cleared, often in a rapid and dramatic way.

HOW TO PERFORM ANIMAL EFT

EFT is easily adapted to remote or proxy (surrogate) use. The technique can be learned in a few minutes. First bring to mind the problem. If it is a large or deep-seated problem, such as a phobia, it is best to focus on one specific aspect of the problem at a time. Instead of a general or large (global) issue like "litter box problem," think of "Fluffy urinates under the table." Think of the problem as a forest: To get rid of the forest, you have to remove individual trees one at a time. Minor problems can often be cleared up with one or two rounds of tapping.

Using EFT on cats is especially easy: You don't even need to tap on the cat. While animals do have meridians and points, the best way to perform EFT on animals is by surrogate or proxy tapping. This means you *tap on yourself* to make the changes happen. Here's how to do it.

① First, think of a phrase or a sentence that describes the problem succinctly and clearly to you. You can say, "Sidney is allergic to chicken," or "Sam keeps pestering me while I'm cooking dinner." Surround the statement of intent with the words, "Even though [name] [problem], I deeply and profoundly love and accept [name]."

② Place the palm of your hand on the Sore Spot. When you can feel the warmth of your hand through your clothes, rub the hand round in a small circle, and say the opening statement, which is the statement of intent inside the framework articulated in step 1.

③ Repeat the opening statement three times, continuously rubbing the Sore Spot.

④ Now choose a shortened version of the opening statement, called the Reminder phrase ("this problem"). Tap with one or two fingers, five to ten times, on the following spots (either side is fine) as you say the statement of intent on each point once.

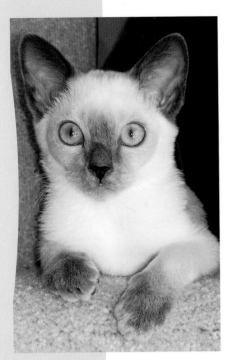

Cat Fanciers' Association's Celestecats Blue Azia, Blue Point Tonkinese, ninth generation raw food-fed kitten

EFT POINTS

EYEBROW: Where the bone behind your eyebrow turns into the bridge of your nose.

CORNER OF THE EYE: On the bone at the outside corner of your eye.

UNDER THE EYE: On the bone just below your eye, in line with your pupil if you look straight ahead.

UNDER THE NOSE: Between your nose and your upper lip.

CHIN: In the indentation between your chin and your lower lip.

UNDERARM: In line with a man's nipples on the side of the body; somewhat lower and toward the back for a woman.

COLLARBONE: In the angle formed by your collarbone and the breastbone.

CROWN: Pat the crown of your head with your flat open hand.

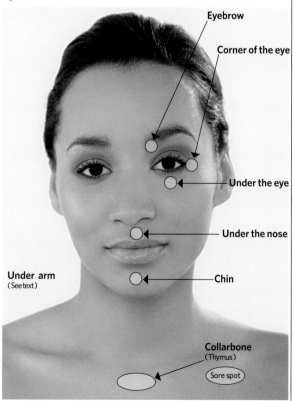

⑤ When you're finished with each round, inhale and exhale deeply. You can continue to repeat the treatment with different statements. Your intuition will often suggest new phrases as you do this. Different statements create different changes, so experiment with many different forms of wording and ways of saying something until you feel comfortable. For chronic physical or behavioral problems, you may need many rounds over a period of time, exploring different aspects.

When you focus your attention on an animal, you *connect* your individual energy systems together. When you then focus your attention on a specific aspect of that energy system (a problem, disease, behavior, etc.), and you change *your* system by tapping on the points, you are also changing the *animal's* system through that connection.

EFT can be applied to a variety of physical and emotional problems, including issues associated with aging. For example, you might work with the following aspects for a cat who sprays urine.

"Even though Fluffy feels a need to spray, I deeply and completely love and accept him."

"Even though Fluffy feels his territory is being threatened..."

"Even though Fluffy doesn't get along with Muffy..."

"Even though I get upset when Fluffy sprays..." (This and similar aspects address the guardian's emotional issues, which can be a significant part of the problem!)

Try EFT on everything: allergies, asthma, relationship problems, past traumas or abuse, pain, disease. (See "Professional Specialists" in Resources on page 178 for contact information to learn more about learning and using EFT.)

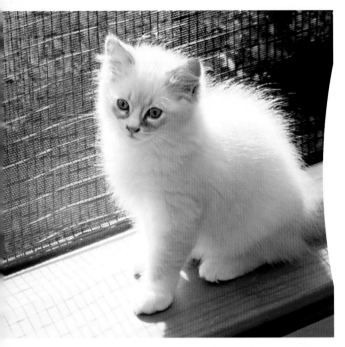

Blue Lynx Point and White Ragamuffin kitten

THE TAPAS ACUPRESSURE TECHNIQUE

The Tapas Acupressure Technique (TAT) is a form of energy work that addresses mental, physical, and emotional traumas. It was developed by Tapas Fleming, a licensed acupuncturist in California. After much research and trial and error, she used a series of points to create her TAT protocol. (See Resources on page 174.)

THE ACTIVE AIR DEVICE

All cellular activities, most importantly the metabolism of oxygen and cell energy production, rely on protein function. It plays a critical role in everything your body does, as well as that of your cat, from movement to digestion to hormone activity. All proteins are water-soluble and only carry out their work in a watery environment.

The Active Air Device (which is made by the Eng3 Corporation; see "Miscellaneous Products" in Resources on page 176 for supplier contact information) improves the cellular environment, thereby enabling the proteins to do their best work. Optimal protein function and cellular rejuvenation help slow the aging process and improve vitality. The device produces a water vapor, which when inhaled influences the fluids within and between cells throughout the body. People use a nasal cannula, plastic tubing with a fitting under the nose, to inhale the vapor. Your cat can get the benefit of the vapor if you place her inside a cat carrier, cover it with a towel, and place the cannula inside (with the nasal fitting cut off, leaving just the tubing). The duration of treatment can be anywhere from five to twenty minutes. Let the cat's behavior guide you. If she gets restless after five minutes, stop and resume later in another session.

Since many illnesses are the result of diminished oxygen utilization and oxidative stress damage such as excessive free radicals, inhaling air from the device improves the body's use of oxygen, oxidative response, and defense against free radical damage. Ultimately, it promotes cell regeneration, protects against premature aging and disease, boosts the immune system, and provides sustainable energy for better overall health and vitality.

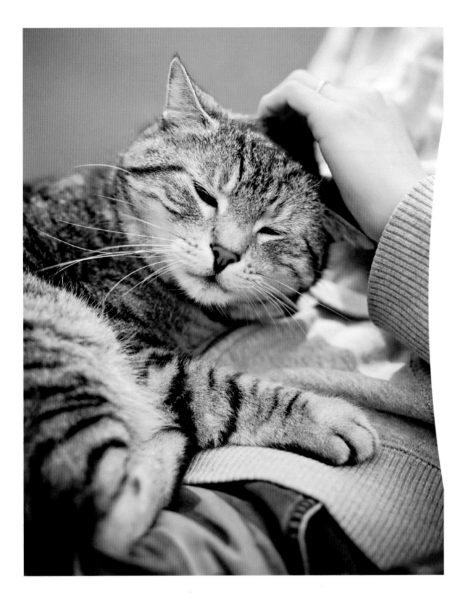

THE BEAUTY OF HANDS-ON HEALING

In addition to all of the benefits outlined in this chapter, hands-on touch therapy of any kind is also an excellent way to help you get closer and strengthen the bonds with your cat. But never force your cat to accept any hands-on work. Try another modality instead. (See chapter 6.) Let your cat tell you how much is okay with him, and for how long.

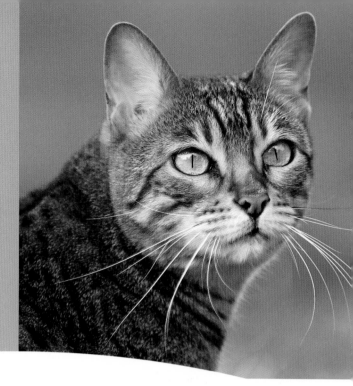

CHAPTER 7

OTHER HEALING MODALITIES AND ANTIAGING THERAPIES

The Tabby-patterned cat usually has an "M" marking on its forehead.

Antiaging and regenerative medicine has become the fastest growing medical specialty in the world. Its goal is to ensure that one's later years are enjoyed in optimum health and well-being. In human medicine, we can fix and even replace body parts that have degenerated; however, these techniques are not readily available for our cats. Certain procedures such as kidney transplantation are available, but they are impractical and unafford-able for all but a very few cats. The future of anti-aging human medicine suggests that we will see such biomedical technologies—such as stem cell therapy, disease detection using cellular biophotons, nanotechnology drug delivery, and even the development of autologous replacement organs—within our lifetimes. One day, we may see these techniques as commonplace in veterinary clinics. Modalities must often first be firmly entrenched in human medicine before they trickle down to our pets. But what can we do in the meantime? As our cats mature and become senior citizens, it is important to support not only their physical well-being (flexibility, eyesight, hearing, energy levels, and general body systems) but their emotional equilibrium as well.

In this chapter, we will look at some of the exciting antiaging therapies that are now being incorporated in veterinary medicine for cats. Also, we will explore energy modalities and other healing approaches that are of interest in our efforts to provide our cats with the healthiest and longest lives possible.

WHAT CAUSES THE SIGNS OF AGING?

Current research points to chronic inflammation as the major cause of many degenerative diseases and other issues of aging, such as liver disease, diabetes, arthritis, and even cancer. However, inflammation is also the body's primary defensive and healing mechanism. Trauma, toxins, allergens, and infectious organisms all trigger inflammation, which allows wounds to heal and viruses and bacteria to be kept in check. The key is to *moderate* inflammation.

Ordinary cellular metabolism is one of the main contributors to the inflammation that constantly waxes and wanes within the body. In the process of burning oxygen to create energy (oxidation), molecules called free radicals are formed. Natural antioxidant molecules in the cells normally scavenge and convert these toxins into less-toxic or non-toxic compounds. When there aren't enough antioxidants available to neutralize them, free radicals will react with and damage other parts of the cell, including fats (a major component of the cell membrane), RNA, and DNA. Accumulated damage can kill the cell, or cause degenerative diseases, including cancer, and other changes associated with aging. When normal inflammation is added to the constant insults the body faces every day from food, water, and air, the normal defenses get overwhelmed, and chronic disease begins.

In all animals, natural antioxidants can be found either in the fatty cell membrane or in the watery cell interior. Because the body can make only a limited amount of its own antioxidants, when external inflammatory stresses are increasing rapidly, it seems sensible to use supplemental antioxidants to support and even boost its free radical-fighting capacity. Scientific evidence demonstrates that such supplements are helpful allies in the battle against aging for both animals and people. However, some natural antioxidants can't be supplemented directly because they aren't effective if taken orally. What we can do is provide the body with abundant building blocks and keep it healthy enough to make plenty of its own.

Not all Supplements are Safe for Cats

Supplements that may work for humans and dogs can be deadly for cats, including the following:

ALPHA LIPOIC ACID: Research shows that it is highly toxic, even lethal, to cats.

ALOE VERA: It contains a latex-like compound that can cause serious irritation in the mouth and gastrointestinal tract if ingested by cats. It is often preserved with sodium benzoate, another toxin.

VINPOCETINE (from the plant *Vinca minor*): It is considered to reduce immune function in cats.

Some advanced supplement formulas include these substances and are well advertised for dogs and cats; however, we advise against their use and suggest you read all labels carefully. Discuss all supplements, their use, and dosages with a veterinarian knowledgeable in clinical nutrition for cats.

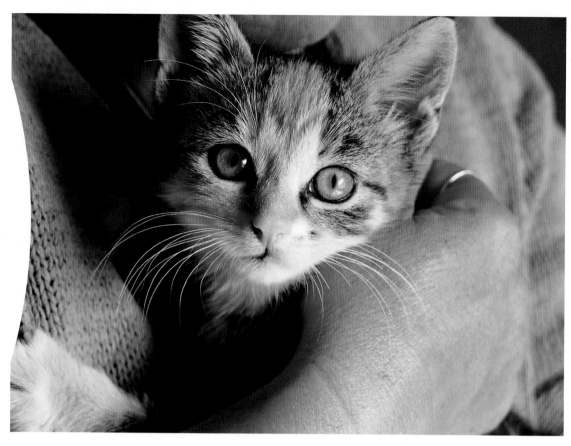

Remember that "natural" does not always equal "safe".

ANTIAGING SUPPLEMENTS

Aside from lifestyle (we already know the benefits and safety of living indoors and being loved and treated as a member of a family) and the genetic hand our pets have been dealt, you can take steps to help your cat live to her full life expectancy. How can you guard against turning on potentially dangerous genes that might have been passed down the line to your cat? The various modalities covered in this book can be used to prevent chronic damage to your cat's body and energy. Are there super supplements for cats as there are for people? The answer is yes; however, they have not been fully tested on cats and must be considered with caution.

When considering antiaging supplements (not including those required to balance the diet, see chapter 4), look for products bearing a seal from the National Animal Supplement Council. These companies have gone through an extensive certification process.

The following supplements have been selected for their superior antiaging properties and general safety. Some have specific benefits for one or more organs or organ systems. However, remember that "natural" does not equal "safe," and any substance can be harmful to any individual cat. We suggest that you discuss these supplements with your holistic veterinarian before adding them to your antiaging regime.

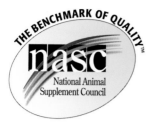

When shopping for antiaging supplements, choose products with this seal from the National Animal Supplement Council if possible.

NOTE: The success of these supplements is contingent on the diet and basic supplementation outlined in chapter 4. Simply giving supplements with commercial pet food from bags and cans is no different from eating cheeseburgers and swallowing vitamins with a soda!

Supplements can be given in the following ways:

- Directly by mouth (Follow dry tablets and capsules with at least 3 ml of purified water, given by syringe.)

- Crush tablets in a mortar and pestle or in a coffee grinder reserved for that purpose and then mix with food or organic broth, which doesn't contain onion or garlic.

- Open capsules and mix the contents with food or organic broth, which does not contain onion or garlic.

- Give liquids by syringe or eyedropper or mixed with onion- and garlic-free food or broth.

Ask your veterinarian for guidance in administering supplements. You'll find doses and associated organ systems in Appendix 1, "Antiaging Supplements for Cats" on page 153.

Stress, the Immune System, and Aging

It's well accepted that both psychological and environmental stress have a negative impact on the immune system. Chronic stress suppresses the immune system, which not only leaves the animal vulnerable to infections, but also reduces the immune system's ability to deal with excess inflammation-causing free radicals. Immune cells produce free radicals as a defense against invading organisms, but they also scavenge and destroy them. If they can't adequately perform that task, accumulated free radicals can damage DNA and play a major role in degenerative diseases of aging, such as arthritis, cognitive dysfunction (senility), and cancer.

Lowering stress, keeping the immune system healthy, and preventing cellular and DNA damage from free radicals and other toxic compounds, are the keys to antiaging for our cats. We can alleviate psychological stress by using flower essences, play therapy, massage, touch, sound, and other stress-relieving methods discussed throughout this book. To minimize the effects of physical and environmental stress, a fresh, raw diet (see chapter 4), supplemented with omega-3 fatty acids and antioxidants, can help keep inflammation in check and maintain the body in a strong, healthy, and youthful state.

GUIDE TO ANTIAGING SUPPLEMENTS

FOR A DOSING SCHEDULE, SEE PAGES 153–155

ACAI: This tropical fruit is loaded with flavonoid antioxidants that may have significant antiaging benefits. It contains amino acids and trace minerals that improve muscle tone and slow down the destructive effects to the skin. It also contains oleic acid, a fatty acid that helps keep cell membranes flexible.

BETA-GLUCANS: These are polysaccharides (complex sugars), usually derived from mushrooms or yeast, with significant immune-boosting power. They are used to stimulate the immune system. While this supplement should not be used continually, it can safely be used for several months when the immune system needs special support, such as while recovering from injury, surgery, or cancer therapy. Medicinal mushroom combinations (using species such as *Reishi*, *Maitake*, *Tremella*, *Poria*, and *Polyporus*), are concentrated sources of beta-glucans without the allergic potential of yeast.

BLUE-GREEN ALGAE (*CYANOBACTERIA*): There are many species of blue-green algae, some of which are beneficial and others highly toxic. Edible blue-green algaes include *Spirulina*, *Dunaliella*, *Heomatoccoccus*, and *Chlorella*. (See "Supplements and Whole Food Products" in Resources on page 174 for supplier information.) These truly are super supplements, packed with amino acids, essential fatty acids, enzymes, and trace minerals.

CAROTENOIDS: This is a large group of antioxidant plant pigments, including the following:

Astaxanthin: These are red plant pigments with superior antioxidant capacity; cats absorb them readily. They are used especially by infection-fighting white blood cells.

Beta-carotene: Although cats cannot convert beta-carotene to vitamin A, they can absorb it, and it may provide significant antioxidant benefits.

Lutein: A yellow or orange pigment found in carrots, squash, and other orange and yellow fruits and vegetables as well as green leafy vegetables such as spinach. Lutein is highly concentrated in the retinas and is important for good vision.

Lycopene: Found most abundantly in tomatoes, lycopene is a fat-soluble red plant pigment with excellent antioxidant and cancer-fighting capabilities.

CARNITINE (*N-ACETYL L-CARNITINE*): An amino acid found primarily in red meat with specific benefits for liver disease and for aging. It improves body composition by decreasing abdominal fat and increasing muscle mass.

CHLOROPHYLL: The plant equivalent of hemoglobin, chlorophyll is a natural gastrointestinal cleanser and detoxifier; it also contains vitamin K, which is crucial for blood clotting. Chlorophyll is loaded with antioxidants, and evidence suggests it has significant anti-cancer properties.

CHOLINE: An essential nutrient, choline is found in liver and eggs. Choline and phosphatidylcholine are components of the cell membrane and are used in the synthesis of neurotransmitters, which are important intercellular messengers. Choline and phosphatidylcholine may help prevent degenerative changes in the brain that lead to senility.

COENZYME Q10: Also known as CoQ10 and ubiquinone, coenzyme Q10 is unique—and powerful—because it stops the inflammatory oxidation process before it begins by helping cells use oxygen more efficiently and produce fewer free radicals. CoQ10 is best absorbed in an oil-based formula; the most bioavailable process is called Q-Gel. It's manufactured by several brands.

COLOSTRUM: Also called "first milk," this is the thin yellowish fluid produced by mammary glands prior to real milk and comprises the first few meals for the newborn. Colostrum is full of antibodies, growth factors, enzymes, immune factors, hormones, and micronutrients; it provides the young with immunity while their own immune systems are still developing. Cows produce large amounts of colostrum, and this is the source for most commercial formulations. It has been used to treat allergies, cancer, colitis, diarrhea, poor wound healing, and many types of infection. Colostrum could be called the first antiaging supplement since it is the first food of all mammal babies.

CURCUMIN: This is the major flavonoid component of turmeric, a mild-tasting yellow spice. It has anti-angiogenic properties, and it is a powerful antioxidant.

VITAMIN E: This is the body's major fat-soluble antioxidant. It is particularly important to supplement with extra vitamin E when feeding oils or fatty meats. It appears that the best choice is a supplement including alpha-tocopherol (what we normally think of as vitamin E) with "mixed tocopherols." This is more likely to come from a natural source.

ECKLONIA CAVA: This kelp extract has been shown to have anti-inflammatory, immunomodulatory, anticancer, and cell protective effects against toxins and radiation. It protects the skin against aging effects, and it has memory-enhancing abilities.

FLAVONOIDS: A large group of antioxidants found in fruits and vegetables, they have antiviral, antiallergic, antiplatelet, anti-inflammatory, antitumor properties. Examples include the following:

Anthocyanadins and proanthocyanadins: These red and blue plant pigments are found in blueberries, blackberries, raspberries, and strawberries.

Vitamin C: Cats make some vitamin C within their bodies, but given the modern stresses of air, light, sound, electromagnetic, and other forms of pollution that we and our pets are exposed to daily, there are clear benefits of adding more to the diet. A vitamin C whole-food complex is ideal, because it contains many other helpful compounds.

Quercitin: This well-studied antioxidant found in apples, grapefruit, grapes, blueberries, and broccoli has unique anticancer properties, and it blocks substances involved in allergies.

SILYMARIN AND SILYBUM: These are extracts of active ingredients of the milk thistle plant, which has been used for centuries to protect and heal the liver, the body's major detoxifying organ. A healthy liver is one of the best defenses against the aging effects of toxins.

GOJI BERRY (*Lycium* spp.): Also called "wolf-berries," goji berries are members of the nightshade family from the valleys of the Himalayas renowned for its long-lived peoples. Goji berries contain a high concentration of antioxidants, including Vitamin C, lutein, and selenium, as well as germanium sesquioxide, an organic mineral complex with significant anti-cancer properties. Known as the "longevity fruit," Goji berries are traditionally used to support kidney and liver function, fortify the bones, and enhance qi (chi), the basic life force.

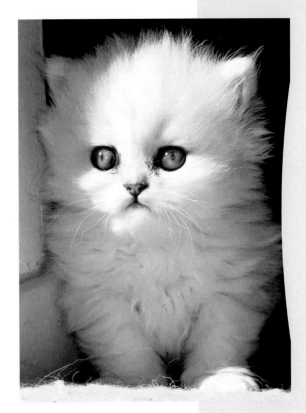

Silver Chinchilla Persian Kitten

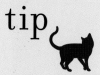

tip

Caution: Safe Dosages Only

Do not experiment with any supplements. Get safe dosages designed for your cat from the chart in the appendix, or from a veterinarian well versed in feline clinical nutrition and the emerging veterinary specialty of antiaging for cats. Avoid products containing sugar and the preservative sodium benzoate. Sugar is unnecessary, and as an empty carb it interferes with insulin metabolism. Sodium benzoate is toxic.

LACTOFERRIN: An antibacterial component of colostrum, lactoferrin is especially useful in treating stomatitis (inflammation of the mouth) in cats.

L-LYSINE: This essential amino acid is a building block for proteins in the body. L-lysine is involved in calcium absorption as well as production of hormones, enzymes, and antibodies. L-lysine is a limiting amino acid in all cereal grains, which may explain why so many cats (many of whom eat grain-based dry food) have problems with upper respiratory herpes virus infections. Supplementing lysine is one treatment for this disease.

MELATONIN: This natural hormone is produced by the pineal gland and also by the eyes and gastrointestinal tract. It regulates circadian rhythms of several biological functions, including the wake/sleep cycle. It has a mild sedating effect and is sometimes prescribed for anxiety. It is also a powerful antioxidant that protects nuclear and mitochondrial DNA. Melatonin may be helpful for cats with chronic kidney disease.

MSM: This is a source of elemental sulfur, the third most abundant element in the body and a component of all connective tissues. Sulfur reserves decrease with age. MSM, besides having its own antioxidant activity, contributes to ongoing maintenance and repair in connective tissues including skin, cartilage, ligaments, and tendons. It is often combined with glucosamine for arthritis and joint pain.

NONI (*Morinda citrifolia*): The tropical noni fruit is reported to have antibacterial, antiviral, antifungal, antioxidant, antitumor, antiparasitic, anti-inflammatory, and immune-enhancing effects. However, many noni juice products are high in sugar and should be avoided.

OLIVE OIL: Monounsaturated olive oil has important antioxidant activity and is able to increase glutathione (one of the body's main natural antioxidants) in the mitochondria.

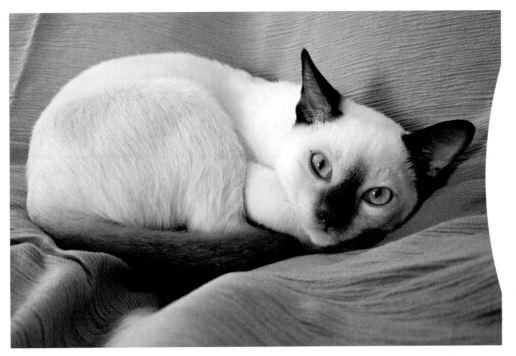

Cat Fancier's Association's Premier Celestecats Matrix, Champagne Point Tonkinese, sixth generation raw food-fed kitten

OMEGA-3 FATTY ACIDS: These anti-inflammatory essential fatty acids are used by every cell in the body, but they are especially critical for the brain, heart, immune system, and skin. The best omega-3s for cats are eicosapentaenoic acid (EPA) and docosahexaenoic acid (DHA), which are found mainly in fish body oil and cod liver oil.

PHENOLS AND POLYPHENOLS: Antioxidants in this group include the flavonoids, as well as compounds found in green tea, olive oil, pomegranates, and cayenne pepper.

PROBIOTICS: These "friendly" bacteria live primarily in the colon and help break down proteins. They include *L. acidophilus*, *Bifidobacterium* spp., and *Enterococcus faecium*. *Enterococcus* appears to be especially important in cats. If a cat or kitten must be on an antibiotic, give probiotics during the course of the drug treatment and for a month afterward. The probiotics replace the friendly bacteria in the intestinal tract that are wiped out by the antibiotic.

SAMe (*S-Adenosyl-L-Methionine*): Pronounced "Sam-ee," this compound is naturally produced in the body, but production wanes with age and certain conditions. Glutathione, one of the body's most important antioxidants, is derived from SAMe. Oral SAMe is used to treat depression, arthritis, and liver disease.

WILLARD WATER: This is also known as Dr. Willard's Water and Catalyzed Altered Water. It acts as a normalizer on all living things not in a healthy state. Willard Water can help assimilate nutrients more efficiently, increase enzyme activity, and strengthen the immune system. It has been very helpful for cats with chronic herpes and conjunctivitis, and it can be used topically for infections. Always dilute it according to the directions.

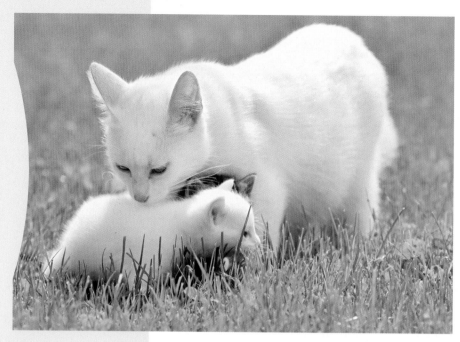

White Domestic Shorthair Cat and Kittens
It's never too soon (or too late) to take steps toward a healthy lifestyle.

tip

Cats Aging Gracefully

Flower essences are very helpful for keeping the mind and spirit youthful and preventing the rigid mental states that often occur as we and our cats age. "Graceful Aging" is a flower essence remedy created by Jean Hofve, D.V.M., (see Resources on page 174) which helps cats cope with the aging process and disperses the unhealthy energy patterns older animals commonly develop that contribute to senility and disease.

Peruvian Salba: An Antiaging Source of Fiber

Salba, the seed of *Salvia hispanica L.*, which is more commonly known as chia, may have benefits for our cats. You can buy it ground, or you can grind it yourself. The seeds originally came in both black and white. But the white-seeded variety was bred separately and named Salba.

The seeds contain antioxidants, calcium, magnesium, protein, and the omega-3 alpha linolenic acid. It can be used for problems such as chronic constipation and/or diarrhea, bloating, and gas, which are conditions found all too often in aging cats raised on commercial pet foods. Salba acts as a colon calmer due to its insoluble fiber content, and it soaks up water because of its soluble fiber content, normalizing stool. It assists with antiaging because it fights free-radical damage, flushes out age-accelerating toxins, and helps build healthy new cells. Salba also helps to maintain healthy skin and coat.

Mix a pinch of the ground seeds into your cat's species-specific meal. Cats don't mind the texture or taste that way.

Treating Cancer Holistically in Cats

Treating cancer requires a carefully planned and executed treatment program designed in conjunction with your veterinary practitioner, including nutrition, energy therapies, and physical support.

Some of the most well-known and widely recommended alternative anticancer therapies include the following herbs:

ESSIAC: This legendary tea is made from burdock root (*Arctium lappa*), Turkey (or Indian) rhubarb (*Rheum palmatum L.*), sheep sorrel (*Rumex acetosella*), and slippery elm bark (*Ulmus fulva*). Essiac, also called Ojibwa Tea, is often used as a general tonic. It is considered safe, but buy it from a reputable source and follow the directions exactly.

HOXSEY FORMULA: This herbal blend contains red clover (*Trifolium pratense*), chaparral (*Larrea tridentata*), licorice root (*Glycyrrhiza glabra*), Oregon grape (*Mahonia aquifolium*), burdock (*Arctium lappa*), sarsaparilla (*Smilax officinalis*), Echinacea (*Echinacea purpurea*), prickly ash bark (*Zanthoxylum clava-herculis*), plus or minus other ingredients depending on the source. Red clover and chaparral can have serious side effects; do not use except under veterinary supervision.

CARNIVORA (Venus fly-trap) (*Dionaea muscipula*): This species of carnivorous plants contains amino acids, quercitin, and other immune modulators that may have cancer-fighting properties.

GERMANIUM: An immune-stimulating trace mineral with a unique ability to correct critical imbalances in the body; it is thought to also have cancer-fighting properties.

GRAVIOLA (*Annona muricata*): Studies in humans have shown promise, especially against multidrug-resistant cancer cell lines.

MISTLETOE (*Viscum album L. Iscador*): The mistletoe plant itself is highly toxic; however, there are preparations or extracts that are thought to stimulate the immune system, kill cancer cells, and help reduce tumor size. It is typically used in conjunction with surgery, chemotherapy, and/or radiation because it may help minimize side effects of these radical treatments. Mistletoe herbal extracts are available, but due to potential toxicity don't use them without close veterinary supervision.

APPLIED KINESIOLOGY

Many holistic veterinarians, clinical nutritionists, and practitioners in energy medicine include methods of Applied Kinesiology (AK) to determine a cat's individual needs. AK is the study of muscles and the relationship of muscle strength to health. AK incorporates functional neurology, anatomy, physiology, biomechanics, and biochemistry with a few bits from acupuncture and massage. Essentially it is a system of manual muscle testing based on the theory that problems can be identified by a muscle weakness in a particular part of the body. George G. Goodheart, D.C., a chiropractor, correlated each large muscle in the body to an organ or organ system. He found that weakness in a muscle may suggest that there is a weakness or disorder in the associated organ. He reasoned that when a nutritional supplement or remedy was held in the subject's hand or held near their body, and the associated muscle "tested strong," that function of the organ would be made strong as well. If it was not the correct remedy, the muscle would test weak.

There are several offshoots of AK, including Contact Reflex Analysis and Quantum Reflex Analysis. Some practitioners also use acupuncture meridians in the protocol.

AK provides the veterinary practitioner with a quick and practical method to test your cat for recommended supplements, remedies, or medication which she deems beneficial for your cat. AK may be included as a complementary diagnostic tool when examining your cat. Your vet may even use it to determine dosages and schedules for various supplements, remedies, or flower essences.

VETERINARY ENERGY MEDICINE

In addition to nutritional support, many devices target the energetic fields in and around us to neutralize damaging radiation and support healing in the body. These can also be considered antiaging since they purport to prevent oxidative cellular damage as well as heal that which is already present. There is less hard science supporting many of these devices, yet thousands of compelling reports from people who have experienced healing for themselves and their pets are hard to ignore. In this section, we provide an overview of the field of energy healing, and we suggest that you discuss the most appropriate therapies for your cat with your holistic veterinarian.

The basic concept behind energy medicine is that all life forms are submerged in the electromagnetic field of the Earth. Additionally, each life form has its own electromagnetic field that, when distorted enough, results in disease. The electromagnetic field of the Earth provides the link between the practitioner and patient during analysis and treatment. It is an ancient axiom that energy follows thought, and thought is transmitted through the energy field of the Earth, allowing the practitioner to attune himself to the patient.

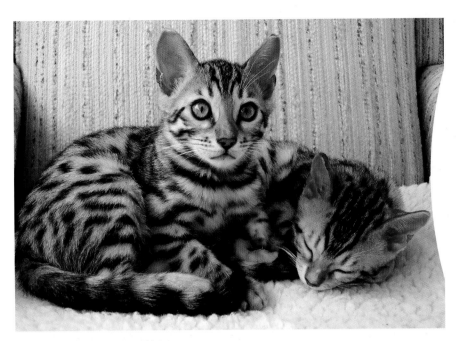

Brown Spotted Tabby Bengal kittens

BIORESONANCE THERAPIES

As quantum physics has proved, matter and energy are one and the same; this is the meaning of Einstein's great equation, E=mc2. As a result, we can influence physical matter by altering its energy fields. Bioresonance, also called bio-energetics, is the field of frequency therapy that seeks to bring the energy fields of two living beings—the practitioner and the patient—into harmony or resonance. Bioresonance instruments are believed to be able to detect pathological dysfunctions in people, plants, and animals before any physical conditions or symptoms arise. There are hundreds of bioresonance techniques and instruments. Some of the more popular ones include: EDS (Electrodermal Screening), Rife therapy, radionics, Intrinsic Data Fields, CoRe, QXCI (Quantum Xeroid Consciousness Interface), Ondamed, SCIO (Scientific Consciousness Interface Operations System), Life-System, Bicom, NES (Nutri-Energetics Systems), SCENAR, Sai Sanjeevini, SE5, SE05, VEGA Tester, Wave Maker, Wave Rider, and VIBE Machine (Vibrational Integrated Bio-photonic Energizer). (See Resources on page 174 for where to find extensive information on many of these techniques.) Veterinarians in the future, using one or more of these devices, and properly trained in these technologies, may be able to recognize potential danger signs, pinpointing and eliminating disease-producing toxins from the body long before they can become destructive. Perhaps one day we'll look back on invasive procedures such as drugs, vaccinations, and surgery as if they were techniques of the Dark Ages. Until then, our best alternative is to stay abreast of developments in human regenerative medicine. The more demand for wellness, life extension, and antiaging breakthroughs, the more our veterinarians will study these subjects and provide this care to our cats.

We suggest caution, careful research, and training before relying on any of these devices for a diagnosis or treatment. Always consult your veterinarian before implementing any of these energy modalities.

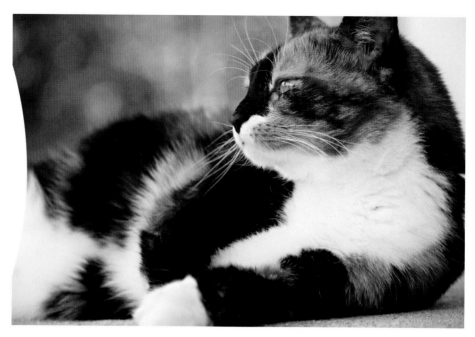

Calico Cats are believed to be good luck in the folklore of many cultures.

TESLA'S PURPLE PLATES

Purple or "positive energy" plates are based on physicist Nikola Tesla's ideas about energy and primary substance, the etheric medium that fills all of space and from which all matter originates. The story behind purple plates is that inventor Ralph Bergstresser worked on the theory with Tesla for twenty years. After Tesla's death, Bergstresser managed to create them by altering the atomic structure in aluminum plates so that a positive energy field surrounds the purple plate. This energy is said to penetrate whatever substance placed on or near it. Advocates of the plates suggest that this energy benefits plants, people, and pets. The plates are thought to hasten healing by returning an injured area, for example, to its normal vibration. Proponents use the plates to raise energy levels and protect against electromagnetic fields (EMFs) in the ambient environment, such as those produced by computers, microwaves and other appliances, and cell phones. You can place purple plates under your cat's bed, food, and water dishes, and you can attach purple disks to the cat's collar. Put a purple disc on your computer to protect against harmful EMFs. (See "Purple Plates" in Resources on page 174 for supplier information.)

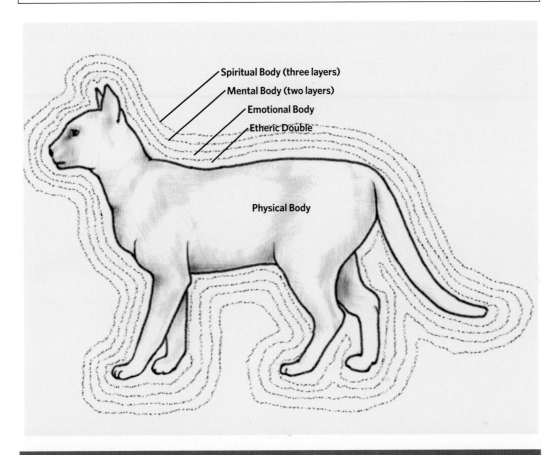

Spiritual Body (three layers)
Mental Body (two layers)
Emotional Body
Etheric Double

Physical Body

THE ETHERIC DOUBLE IS THE NEAREST NONPHYSICAL LEVEL.

AURAS, CHAKRAS, AND COLORS

An aura is an electromagnetic energy field that surrounds, encompasses, and permeates all living things; it includes the being's physical structure as well as its energetic outer layers. It is made up of four bodies outside the physical body: the etheric body (where some suggest our past life experiences may be stored), the emotional body, the mental body (two layers: higher and lower), and the spiritual body (three layers: higher, middle, and lower). The colors of an aura vary depending upon the condition of the being. Anyone can learn to see auras; there are also professional readers and even cameras that can photograph them.

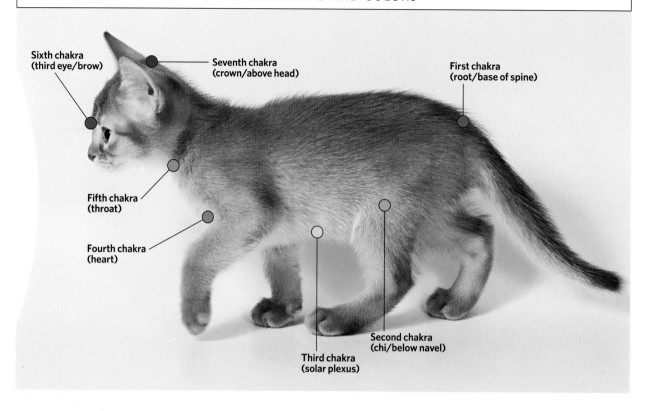

Sixth chakra (third eye/brow)

Seventh chakra (crown/above head)

First chakra (root/base of spine)

Fifth chakra (throat)

Fourth chakra (heart)

Second chakra (chi/below navel)

Third chakra (solar plexus)

The chakras are energy centers aligned along a spiral column in the etheric double; energy is absorbed from the surrounding air and brought through the chakras into the physical body. The Vedas, ancient texts of India, contain the first known reference to chakras. The chakras are considered to be spinning wheels of light energy. (Chakra means "wheel" in Sanskrit.) Various spiritual schools have different systems of identification for the chakras, but a widely accepted version identifies seven major chakras, beginning with the first, or root, chakra, located at the base of the spine and moving up the body to the seventh, or crown, chakra, located a few inches above the top of the head. (There are also five minor chakras, at the hands and feet/paws and the hollow at the base of the skull, where the brain meets the spine. It is said that as we spiritually evolve, new chakras will emerge.)

A specific color is associated with each chakra and can be used to stimulate, sedate, or balance the chakras and their associated organs. The use of light and color in healing dates from ancient times. In Ayurvedic medicine, it is believed that there are cycles that are the most conducive for certain activities. In Chinese medicine, yang and yin symbolize light and dark. It is of utmost importance to honor our daily cycles of light turning into darkness, as our moon travels around our planet and our planet travels around our sun. (See Appendix 2: Astromedicine for Cats, page 156, for the correlation of colors to the sun signs of the zodiac.)

FIRST CHAKRA (root/base of spine)

Red stimulates the immune system by building up the blood and helps with detoxification. This color fights tumors, has an antiviral effect, and relates to the reproductive system and the procreative imperative to survive. Cats with feline leukemia and compromised immune systems should be surrounded by the color red as much as possible.

SECOND CHAKRA (chi/below navel)

Orange is an appetite stimulant and a lung builder. It depresses the parathyroid glands, and it stimulates the thyroid as well as the mammary glands in the production of milk. Qi (chi) emanates from this chakra.

THIRD CHAKRA (solar plexus)

Yellow stimulates the gastrointestinal system and helps keep hormones in balance. It's also beneficial for the liver, gallbladder, kidneys, and for diabetes and hard chronic tumors. The fear/fight/flight mechanism originates here.

FOURTH CHAKRA (heart)

Green stabilizes energy and is a bronchodilator. It's beneficial in the treatment of infections. Many believe that love emanates from the heart chakra. Pink is the secondary color of the heart chakra.

FIFTH CHAKRA (throat)

Blue aids in the healing of third-degree burns, scratches, sores, and infections. It's beneficial for all fevers that respond quickly when used in conjunction with holistic remedies. Blue is a very cooling and sedating color. The related color turquoise soothes irritations, inflammation, and itching. It helps induce sleep, and it should follow green in treating all infections. It is known as the chakra of self-expression.

SIXTH CHAKRA (third eye/brow)

Indigo worn around the neck helps stabilize the thyroid if an animal has a hyperthyroid condition. The third eye chakra is best known for providing living things with intuition and instinct.

SEVENTH CHAKRA (crown/above head)

Violet increases the white blood cell count, stimulates the spleen, and is a color for high spiritual attainment in humans.

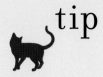

Using Color with Cats

Color therapy for cats can be provided with cuddle beds, blankets, and throws in appropriate colors for various conditions that arise from time to time. If your cat will tolerate wearing a kerchief around her neck; try keeping several different colors on hand.

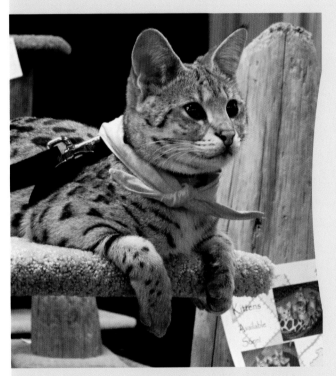

Brown Spotted Tabby Savannah

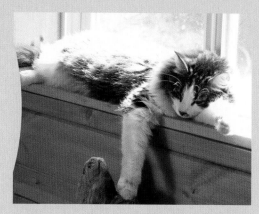

Black and White Domestic Longhair

Light Toxicity

When we don't sleep in sync with seasonal light exposure, we alter our biological rhythms that control hormones and neurotransmitters determining appetite, fertility, and mental and physical health. By relying on artificial light to extend our days, we fool our bodies into living in a perpetual state of summer. Anticipating the scarce food supply and forced inactivity of the coming winter, our body begins storing fat and slowing the metabolism to sustain us through months of hibernation and hunger that never arrive. Our cats, when they took the evolutionary step of crossing our thresholds to live with us, also suffer from light toxicity when we are out of sync with our natural daily rhythms.

All animals are extremely sensitive to natural light and dark rhythms, including humans. There is a strong case for all animals to sleep in the summer months between 10:00 p.m. (2200 hours) and 7:00 a.m. (0700), and starting at the Autumn Equinox between 9:00 p.m. (2100) and 6:00 a.m. (0600). Our early ancestors obeyed these seasonal rules by honoring the seasons and their natural rhythm of light and dark. Our bodies generate a cascade of protective chemicals, including those that help prevent cancer, obesity, diabetes, and depression, to name but a few, only when we sleep deeply with no interference from any light whatsoever, including the LEDs on electronic equipment, digital clocks, night lights, and light leaks from outside. We desperately need a true black night sleeping experience. The ramifications of not honoring this rule are enormous for our own health as well as that of our cats. They also suffer from our addiction and abuse of light.

Studies suggest that even tiny light leaks (0.2 lux), as little as a single candle flame, adversely affect our own health and that of our cats. If light leakage and subsequent lack of melatonin promotes tumor growth, could the use of light after dark actually be one of the causes of cancer in people and their pets? (For suppliers of full-spectrum lighting, see "Full-Spectrum Lighting" in Resources on page 174.)

CRYSTALS AND HEALING

Crystals are solidified minerals created when water combines with an element under certain conditions of pressure, temperature, and energy. Crystals don't interact directly with the physical body, but rather with the fundamental energy system that creates and support the body, and connects it with the mind and emotions. The physical body exists only by virtue of energy; we get energy from food, water, air, and the Earth itself. In conjunction with the mind, crystals can create all types of healing that manifest in the physical body.

Crystals pick up the energies of the people and places where they have been, and they accumulate both positive and negative vibrations. Negative energies can also come from electromagnetic radiation from televisions, cell phones, and computers.

When you first acquire your crystals, you should always cleanse them as soon as you can. Here are a few possibilities.

🌀 Smudge the crystals with sage and sweetgrass or your favorite incense.

🌀 Rinse crystals in running water. Check first to make sure that your type of crystal can tolerate water.

🌀 Set your crystal in or on sea salt or Himalayan salt. Check first to make sure that your type of crystal can tolerate salt.

🌀 Set your crystal in or on a large quartz crystal, citrine, or amethyst cluster.

🌀 Cleanse your crystal with flower essences or Reiki.

When the crystals are cleared, "fill them" with your positive intentions to keep them from reabsorbing negative energy. Recleanse them after use.

Tumbled or polished stones seem to open up and increase energy and may easily be used under seat cushions, cat beds, and birthing beds; or place one in the water bowl to energize your cat's purified water.

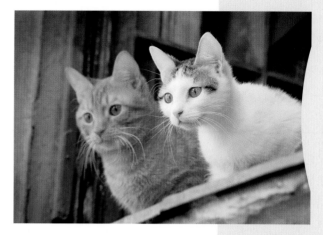

Domestic Shorthairs

HEALING WITH SOUND

The same everyday noises that bombard us from the moment we awake also bombard our cats, but it sounds three times louder to them! While cats miss out on some of the lower sounds, they hear higher sounds than even dogs do (up to 60,000 hertz). Cats' immune systems, like ours, can break down amid the unnatural influences of the modern world. Soothing sounds can enhance their feeling of well-being, just as they do ours. Listening to music or healing sounds may augment other healing therapies. Cats naturally use sound for healing themselves. Their purring is in the range of healing frequencies.

Sound has been used for millennia for healing. Tibetan bells, crystal bowls, Gregorian and Buddhist chants, mantras, and the most natural and powerful, "over toning" (vocal harmonics with the human voice) are among the tools still used today to achieve spiritual realization and healing. They can be used for healing our cats as well. (See "Music" in Resources on page 174 for suppliers' contact information.)

Music reduces stress, and you and your cats can experience many benefits by listening together. Animal facilities from shelters to dairy barns use music to keep animals calm, healthy, and productive. Cats respond quite favorably to Mozart. Perhaps this can be explained by a study which found that listening to ten minutes of a Mozart piano sonata improved the scores of college students in a test of abstract reasoning. The researchers believe the music stimulated brain cell activity. You might want to leave your radio on a classical music station to keep your cats content while you are out.

Whatever soothing sounds or music you choose should be enjoyed by not only you but your cats, too.

MAGNETIC THERAPY

The oldest form of physical therapy known to humankind, magnetic therapy dates back to 420 B.C. when Hippocrates used magnets to treat jaundice and hernias. Biochemistry has historically overshadowed biophysics. As this emphasis shifts, medicine will undergo rapid change, such as illustrated by the use of magnets in healing.

A magnet is an object, such as a piece of iron or steel, that is charged with an electromagnetic field. Magnets possess the ability to attract certain substances, such as iron. Each magnet has two poles, north (yin/green) and south (yang/red).

Many practitioners who use magnets believe that exposure to the north pole of a magnet slows down the processes of the body, relaxes the muscles, decreases blood pressure, decreases growth of abnormal cells, treats fractures by decreasing acidity (allowing bones to heal fast), sedates the nervous system, decreases the growth of bacteria and viruses, decreases inflammation, and assists in the healing of burns. In addition, exposure to north decreases the white blood cell count and increases the red blood cell count, which when done just after birth increases the life span by decreasing protein metabolism and thus increasing intelligence. (Note: The south pole increases intelligence when used just *before* birth).

Practitioners believe that exposure to the south pole increases cell growth, stimulates the production of endorphins, and increases the size of tumors, the growth of bacteria and viruses, the amount of sodium in the body, and the level of acidity. If used on a fracture, it increases healing time. Never use the south pole to treat cats who have active infections. And do not use the south pole over the head, as it may create abnormal behavior and increase inflammatory reactions in the body by increasing the white blood cells.

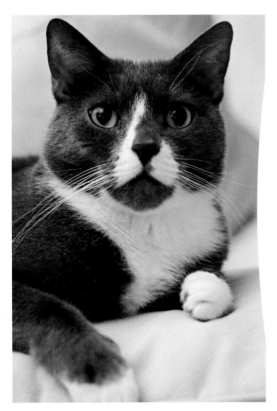

Blue and White Domestic Shorthair
Cat fanciers refer to gray cats as "Blue."

THERAPEUTIC USES FOR MAGNETS

Animals suffering from afflictions as diverse as arthritis and hyperactivity may benefit from magnetic therapy. You can buy many versions of neutrally polarized magnetic pads for animals to lie upon. Some report that they relieve pain and inflammation, stimulate tissues, increase circulation, increase oxygen to the tissues, and facilitate rehabilitation. Clear the use of any form of magnetic therapy with your vet or holistic practitioner before using it on your cat.

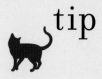

tip

Far Infrared Heat

Pain from injury and/or aging affects cats as much as humans. Far infrared pet pads or pet beds contain infrared heating elements that emit deep-penetrating, far infrared rays. These rays may promote blood flow, which can reduce inflammation and provide pain relief for cats suffering from strains, arthritis, muscle pain, or joint pain. The pads provide extra warmth and help in the recovery process following surgery or other treatments.

Try using a far infrared cat bed for birthing mothers and kittens because maintaining their 101°F (38°C) body temperature is of critical importance to building their immune systems. Older cats enjoy the warmth, too, and it encourages them to stay off your electronic equipment! (See Resources on page 174.)

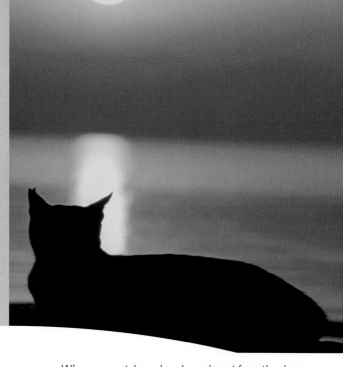

SAYING GOOD-BYE TO THE ONES WE LOVE

When one watches a loved one depart from the shore, another welcomes them on the opposite shore.

The loss of a cat can be an agonizing experience. To most animal lovers, our animal companions are every bit as important as members of our human family. People who have suffered the loss of their cats usually have other family members and or pets who are also grieving the loss.

The question that most often arises is: Do we wait, or do we adopt a cat or kitten to help fill this empty void? Certainly a kitten or an adult cat can be there to help and comfort the grieving. But even more than that, when one is used to loving their pet, it's very difficult to not have a recipient upon whom to lavish this flow of love because our love doesn't die when our loved ones do. Adopting a kitten or adult cat from an animal shelter may be the answer. With so many cats in shelters in desperate need of homes and people to love them, the ideal way to help the grieving process and to prevent their needless death is to bring home one of these babies. These adoptions are beneficial to both the adopter and adoptee.

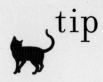

COMMUNICATING WITH YOUR SICK OR AGING CAT

The decisions that plague us at the end of our pets' lives are heavy burdens to bear. For instance, is it too late to seek alternative healing therapies when the animal has been through so much? Should we choose euthanasia (a humane death by injection), or permit our animals to endure until the end? If you choose not to euthanize, you'll want to provide hospice-type care to make sure your cat remains as comfortable as possible.

Ultimately, you and your animal friend need to make these choices together. Now is the most important time for spiritual work: meditation, prayer, and nonverbal communication. You'll receive guidance when your heart and mind are open. Do what you feel is best, but please make sure you are truly considering your cat's best interests and not just your own needs or inability to let go. Animals have their own paths and their own spiritual journeys. When the end is near, the best thing you can do for them is to release them. Tell them out loud that it's okay for them to pass on. This will help you accept it, and it will help them follow the path ahead. Flower essences can be extremely helpful to ease this transition. (See "Flower Essences" in chapter 5.)

Some animal communicators and psychics feel that animals reincarnate in tandem with their human companions and with each other. The closer the interspecies bonding, the more likely and more frequent such reincarnation is to occur. Some even believe the species are interchangeable. Metaphysicians often recommend that you tell your animal companion you understand that they wish to leave this body, and that you will welcome them in their new one, so their spirit may continue its bond with you.

Planning Ahead

Consider making arrangements for your pets in your will or with your loved ones in the event of your death. There have been many cases where pets have come to tragedy when their people died without leaving instructions for their care. (See Pet Loss in Resources on page 174 for books offering more information on planning for such a situation.)

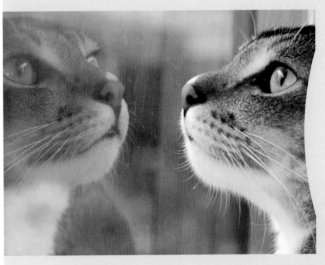

Think ahead; don't leave your cat's future uncertain.

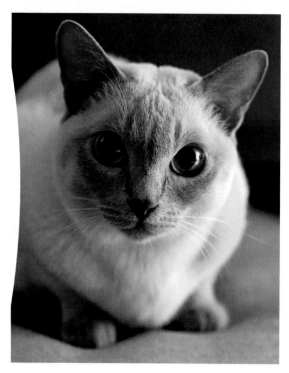

Cat Fanciers' Association's Champion Celestecats China Doll Rose, Platinum Mink Tonkinese, fifth generation raw food-fed cat

MOURNING

The time needed to grieve is personal for everyone. However, it is quite necessary to work through the process, because denial is even more painful, if not truly harmful, in the long run. One way to think about this is to visualize a flight of stairs in front you. Place apathy on the first step, grief on the second, then continue up the stairs to fear, anger, and pride, then allow three more steps at the top of your flight; courage, acceptance, and peace. You might ask yourself which step you currently find yourself standing upon, as these are the most likely steps that one in a healing process must climb to reach the goal of peace. It is often difficult to move from one step to the next as we find ourselves getting stuck.

LETTING GO

Grasp an object, such as a pen, in your hand and squeeze it as hard as you can, and then turn your hand over and open your hand. Just let the object fall; release it. If you can imagine releasing a feeling, such as anger with this much ease, the process becomes simple, even elegant. Move through each one of the steps of grieving in your own time and release these emotions. Flower remedies are also helpful at times like these. (See chapter 5.) You may select one or more that resonate appropriately to the feeling you and your animal companions are experiencing.

Many people do not have anyone with whom they can share this type of loss. Family and friends may not understand the depth of feelings they're experiencing. A pet loss or grief service or therapy group may be the answer. (See "Grief Recovery Institute" in Resources on page 179 for contact information.)

LISTENING TO YOUR HEART

You might view death as a departure on a great ship. Just as the ship sails away from us, and we wave good-bye from the shore, at the same time someone waits on the other side, waving hello. Our animals make this journey with grace if we only allow them this dignity, which is their birthright.

Sometimes euthanasia is the best option, particularly when the last days of an illness are likely to involve suffering, or if treatment will be painful or lengthy, with little hope for full recovery. Quality of life is an issue that veterinarians are taught to consider, but occasionally the enthusiasm for a new chemotherapy drug or surgical technique may override common sense.

Before you allow your beloved animals to be drugged, poked, prodded, or surgically explored, communicate with them and try to ascertain what they want. If they are ready to cross over to the realms of light, the most loving gift is to support them in that journey, whether by euthanasia or supportive hospice care to, allow them to go on their own.

As with living, we can learn so much from our animal friends about death and dying. They seem to view it as a natural progression. It's so very difficult to watch the ones we love leave their physical bodies, and I'm sure they're sad to leave us just as we're sad to lose them. But finally, after we grieve and say farewell, we must concentrate on taking care of the living. We keep our love for the pets who have moved on safely tucked in our hearts. It may be cliché to say that time heals all wounds, as we all carry the scars of those wounds, but somehow we find the strength in their honor to carry on and keep loving, grateful for having had this special being in our lives.

We've been changed permanently by living with our animals. In that way, they live forever in how we interact with the world. Animals, and humans for that matter, may not be of this Earth but could quite possibly be souls that have chosen to use this planet as their setting for a spiritual experience in a physical body. Animals may not operate in the same complicated way as humans but rather participate in life through nature. They are not lesser beings, just different.

MOVING ON

I'm often approached by people who are ready to move forward and bring a new kitten or cat home but want the exact same type of cat as the one they have just lost—down to the sex and color. I always try to steer these people to a rescue facility first. However, many people who have lived with a particular breed simply wish to have another, and they cannot be dissuaded. I explain that there will never be another animal like the one they have just lost, and that it's futile to try and replace him or her. I guide them gently, if the rescue approach fails, to pick a different sex and a different color. It's a little easier to adjust to the differences in personality if the looks are a little different, too. Be fair to the new spirit and embrace the new cat or kitten's uniqueness. When I lost a beloved cat companion, another breeder gave me a cat who could have been my cat's twin. Every time I looked at her, all I could think of was, "you are not my darling girl." No matter how badly I wanted her to be the new version of the cat I lost, it just never happened. I found her a new home with someone who could love her for herself, and not who and what I wanted her to be.

CROSSING THE RAINBOW BRIDGE

Having bred cats for the past sixteen years, one would think I would have toughened up by now. On the contrary, I always cry when I lose a cat, especially a newborn kitten. There never seems to be enough time to spend with these precious little spirits, or the ones you've had the pleasure of raising well into elder years. I have been blessed with friends and clients who love their animal companions as I do and can truly empathize with me. It's even a common occurrence today to receive a sympathy card from your vet when one of your beloved animal companions passes. Often times, the "Rainbow Bridge" poem is offered as support in this time of need. Consider sharing this poem with someone you know who has lost a pet (see page 173).

CONCLUSION

THE FUTURE OF HOLISTIC CAT CARE

We hope you have enjoyed our travels through the world of holistic and antiaging health care for cats as much as Dr. Jean and I have enjoyed being your tour guides. I trust you can feel our passion and excitement for this ever-expanding field, which has become one of the fastest growing areas of health care. We may not have all the tools necessary for cat life-extension at our fingertips, but we have shared with you many ways to provide optimum health for cats until the fullness of these various technologies are realized and readily available.

Cat Fanciers' Association's Premier Celestecats Matrix, Champagne Point Tonkinese, six generation raw food-fed cat

It is never too late to take steps toward a healthier lifestyle for your cat. The following steps are simple; note how similar they are to what we require for our own health and well being.

① Exercise (For cats, we use play therapy.)

② Detoxification and chemical avoidance. (Substitute safe, natural products.)

③ Nutrition and supplementation (Feed species-specific, organic, homemade food.)

④ Safe, effective alternative therapies to conventional drugs and surgery

⑤ Deep, restful sleep.

And last but not least, is the hope for future veterinary therapy.

⑥ Bio-identical/bio-memetic hormone replacement therapy for spayed and neutered pets.

MOTHER NATURE'S ROLE

When it comes to Mother Nature, there is no such thing as antiaging. When Mother Nature thinks our reproductive days are over, she figures it is time to get rid of us and make us part of the food chain. That's what happens out there in the wild. Using protocols such as bio-identical/ bio-mimetic hormones may help us fool Mother Nature in a good way. We hope to see natural hormone replacement options for our spayed and neutered cats in the near future. This is our next big project!

Today there seems to be so much emphasis on inherited disease and DNA driving the scientific community. So often, we are made to feel helpless about our lot in life and that of our pets as well. When we take proper care of ourselves and our pets, it just may be possible to overwrite our genetics. This concept is now referred to as epigenetics, the stable and heritable changes in gene expression that are not attributable to DNA sequence. It is an extremely active area in scientific research today. This makes the tools in this book invaluable, because they may provide a way to avoid switching on potentially dangerous genes, by getting back to the natural order of life. In practice, we become the caretaker of our own genome, as what we do and what we experience in our lives will be passed down to all the generations that follow us and our companion animals when they are used in breeding programs such as mine. Everything we all eat, experience, and think—even our traumas—encode above our genome and are passed down generation after generation. Emotions and environment affect our cats' gene function. Many of these factors are within our control, so it's up to us to to provide the components our cats need to function at a higher, healthier level.

What's on the horizon? Could immortality for human beings be just around the corner? If it is, what can we adapt from human antiaging for our cats to help accomplish this goal for them, too? Could we, through the protocols suggested here, keep ourselves going long enough to make it till the coming biotechnology revolution, which may be able to turn on and off many disease processes, as well as aging? Could our bodies and brains be rebuilt on a molecular level? Will Dr. Jean and I inspire some young vet students to bring this incredible world of possibilities to our cats? If just one of our readers is in vet school at the moment, who knows, he or she may become one of the leaders in antiaging veterinary medicine in the future.

POSITIVE THINKING

It is incredibly important to be steadfastly positive and not allow the negativity and fear we all encounter in our daily lives to prevail. We are what we eat and also what we think! All of us living things are the sum total of all that we believe. Do you ever wonder why what you fear the most often seems to happen, as if it were inevitable? In a way, it was. All life is vibration, and your fear vibrations attract more of the same, until what you were thinking appears. This works for both positive and negative thoughts, so it really is important to accentuate the positive! Practice confidence and positivity, and you'll find it spilling over into every aspect of your life. It takes a real transformation of consciousness to accomplish this shift.

Now is the time to take back the responsibility for our health and that of our cats! We would never be so narrow-minded as to deny completely the usefulness of allopathic Western medicine, but we must make sure that we exhaust every natural method available before we risk the use of drugs or surgery. And when we must resort to using allopathic methods of treatment, we must

take advantage of the many protocols offered in this book to help the body repair from whatever toll they have taken. We've learned recently that even antibiotic use, especially repeated prescriptions, is associated with increased risk of certain cancers. We must learn to help the body heal itself and only turn to drugs and surgery when absolutely necessary to save one's life.

Share this book, as well as your insights and concerns, with your health care providers. This partnership will benefit you, them, and your cat. You may be surprised at how open to new ideas your providers are. But if they're not, the decision about whether to use holistic care still belongs to you.

We are committed to continuing our journey and sharing our findings. Visit our website (www.celestialpets.com) for updates on new advances in veterinary medicine and holistic therapies and even new products we find that might be helpful. Join our email list, and we'll keep you informed.

I personally extend my invitation to all of our readers to be in touch with us through www.celestialpets.com. We can help guide you to reliable resources for acquiring kittens and/or cats for rescue, purchase or adoption, associations involved in the registry of pedigreed cats and how to find cat shows and agility competitions. You will find more information about Celestial Pets and many of the companies, books, activities and practitioners we recommend in Resources on page 174.

Celestial Pets also offers Clinical Nutrition Services to personally work with you through consultation and provide a customized clinical nutrition protocol for your cat. This protocol may then be shared with your vet in order to enlist him as a partner in every aspect of wellness. We look forward to getting to know you and your cat personally!

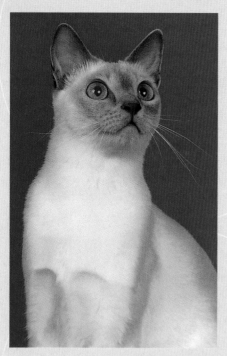

The International Cat Association's Supreme Grand Champion (Alter) Sonham's Romeo of Celestecats, Platinum (Lilac) Point Tonkinese, first generation raw

Bio-Identical and Bio-Mimetic Hormones for Cats:

A POSSIBILITY FOR THE FUTURE

T.S. Wiley, author of *Sex, Lies, and Menopause* and *Lights Out*, is the creator of the Wiley Protocol, an extremely popular, bio-identical/bio-mimetic hormone replacement therapy for people. The Wiley Protocol is my personal choice for my own antiaging regime. When I raised the issue of lack of hormones in our spayed and neutered cats, Wiley expressed her concern that, as necessary as it may be to reduce pet overpopulation, removing their reproductive organs may be shortening cats' lives and accelerating their disease state. She said, "The solution to this problem is legitimate hormone replacement to restore their psychoneuroimmuno-logical endocrine function."

Spaying and neutering is still the best means for decreasing pet over-population and preventing the diseases described earlier. But, this is also a political issue, and I'm addressing our cats' health and longevity. Are there issues that we are not addressing in veterinary medicine as a result of removing those important reproductive organs and hormones? There is a significant body of research showing that spaying and neutering dogs may have a detrimental effect in terms of several types of cancer and other degenerative diseases. Some of these findings may apply to cats. However it is not politically correct to talk about that.

In the wild, when animals are no longer reproducing, they tend to develop aging changes and disease, slowing them down until they starve or become prey to a predator. Mother Nature usually removes the reproductively unfit.

That is why I am proposing the bio-identical/bio-mimetic hormone hypothesis for cats. A bio-identical hormone protocol for our spayed and neutered cats might be an appropriate antiaging therapy for them as well. Perhaps without their reproductive organs, cats suffer from a kind of "cat menopause" (or, for males, andropause). There are hormone replacement protocols for women who have had hysterectomies. What about bio-identical hormones for our animal companions after they have been surgically altered to address the side effects of this procedure? Because our cats can't verbally convey extremely subtle symptoms, are we and our veterinarians missing something critically important?

I stumbled across this idea because of my own use of rhythmic transdermal bio-identical/bio-memetic hormone creams. My spayed female cats came into raging heat from coming into contact with the cream on my arms. (Veterinarians and pharmacists have seen quite a few similar cases.) These symptoms, however, seemed to balance out after I was on bio-identical hormone therapy after about three to six months. Now, to be safe, I wear long sleeves after I use my creams and wash my hands thoroughly. The two creams used most often are estradiol, which builds the lining of the uterus, and progesterone, which causes the uterus to shed its lining. There is also bio-identical testosterone and DHEA, as well as thyroid. Such creams are used in a particular order on particular days that mimic the natural pulsed rhythms of these hormones to achieve their effects.

Subsequently, I posed the question to T.S. Wiley about natural hormones for both spayed females and neutered males. She believes we can come up with a rhythmic protocol for them in the near future; one which would not cause them to revert to the behavior patterns we find so difficult to live with, such as heat cycling and/or territorial marking. Having bred cats for sixteen years, I know all too well the downside to that! Our website will offer updates on this topic as well as other valuable information in the future. (See "Supplements and Whole Foods" in Resources on page 174.)

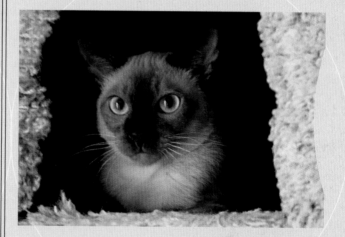

Cat Fanciers' Association's Celestecats A Tango Rose, Natural Mink Tonkinese, eleventh generation raw food-fed cat

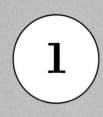

APPENDIX

1

HEALTH REFERENCE TOOLS

TOXIC FOODS, HERBS, AND PLANTS

The following is a list of especially dangerous foods, herbs, and plants for cats:

- Aloe *(Aloe Vera)*
- Amaryllis *(Hippeastrum)*
- Avocado *(Persea gratissima)*
- Azalea *(Rhododendron sp.)*
- Bamboo *(Phyllostachys sp.)*
- Black walnut *(Juglans nigra)*
- Bulbs (all types)
- Cherries *(Prunus Serotina)*
- Chives *(Allium Schoenoprasum)*
- Dumb cane *(Dieffenbachia maculata)*
- Fruit seeds, kernels and pips

- Garlic *(Allium sativum)*
- Grapes, raisins, grape seeds *(Vitis vinifera* sp.)
- Hemlock (all) *(Conium* spp.)
- Holly berry *(Ilex aquifolium)*
- Hyacinth *(Hyacinthus orientalis)*
- Hydrangea *(Macrophylla acuminate)*
- Iris *(Iris versicolor)*
- Ivy (all) *(Hedera helix)*
- Lilies *(Liliaceae)*
- Marigold *(Calendula)*
- Marsh marigold *(Caltha palustris)*
- Milkweed *(Asclepias syriaca)*
- Mistletoe *(Viscum album)*
- Mushrooms
- Nightshades (green, raw or sprouts): eggplant, peppers, potatoes, tobacco, tomatoes
- Nutmeg *(Myristica fragrans)*
- Oleander *(Nerium oleander L.)*

TOXIC DRUGS AND SUPPLEMENTS

The following is a list of especially dangerous drugs and supplements for cats.

- Acetaminophen (Tylenol)
- Alpha lipoic acid
- Aspirin (Use only under direction and supervision of a veterinarian.)
- Ibuprofen (Motrin)
- Naproxen sodium (Aleve)

ANTIAGING SUPPLEMENTS FOR CATS (DOSING SCHEDULE)

The following chart lists specific antiaging supplements for cats described in chapter 7. Doses are given as total per day. If your cat has one or more conditions that you wish to address, do not give more than is recommended for any one condition. For example, if you are giving glucosamine sulfate for both joints and urinary tract, do not double the dose; just give 250 milligrams per day. Because cats are notoriously difficult to supplement, supplements are listed in order of importance. If you can only get one or two supplements into the cat, choose the ones at the top. Always work with your veterinarian to establish exact doses for your cat and to monitor progress. Stop all supplements if condition worsens or if unusual symptoms occur, and contact your veterinarian immediately.

SYSTEM	CONDITIONS	SUPPLEMENTS	DOSE (Per day unless noted)
Whole body		Omega-3 fatty acids	300 to 600 milligrams DHA/EPA
		Probiotics	1 to 5 billion CFU/day. Should include *Enterococcus spp.* Give ¼ to ½ human dose per meal
		Digestive enzymes	As directed, or ½ human dose per meal
		Mixed antioxidants	⅛ human dose each
		Blue-green algae	1 to 3 capsules
		Vitamin E	50 to 200 IU
		Vitamin C	50 to 100 milligrams
		Beta-glucans	50 milligrams
		Colostrum	200 milligrams twice a day
		Noni	1 teaspoon once or twice a day
		Acai	100 milligrams
		Goji	50 milligrams per pound of body weight
Immune system	Asthma, allergies, cancer	Omega-3 fatty acids	300 to 600 milligrams DHA/EPA
		Blue-green algae	1 to 3 capsules
		Mixed antioxidants	⅛ human dose each
		Beta-glucans Turmeric/curcumin	50 milligrams Turmeric powder ¼ teaspoon per meal; curcumin 100 milligrams per meal

SYSTEM	CONDITIONS	SUPPLEMENTS	DOSE (Per day unless noted)
		Astaxanthin	10 milligrams
Blood		Chlorophyll (fat-soluble extract)	1 to 3 drops
Eyes	Herpes conjunctivitis	L-lysine	1,000 milligrams per day for 5 days to treat flare-ups; 250 milligrams per day as preventative
		Aeura herpes formula (homeopathic)	Dissolve 1 tablet in 1 ounce (30 ml) water, give 3 to 5 drops twice a day
		Willard Water	2 ounces (60 ml) per gallon of drinking water
	General vision	Omega-3 fatty acids	300 to 600 milligrams DHA/EPA
Mouth		Omega-3 fatty acids	300 to 600 milligrams DHA/EPA
		Lactoferrin	200 to 300 milligrams twice a day
		Beta glucans	50 milligrams
		Quercitin	¼ to ⅛ of the human dose or 200 milligrams
Liver		Livaplex	1 capsule divided into meals
		Milk thistle/silybum/silymarin/marin	80 percent silymarin extract 25 to 50 milligrams divided among meals; marin 25 milligrams
		SAMe	200 milligrams in enteric-coated tablet; give on empty stomach
		L-carnitine	250 milligrams
		Chlorophyll (fat-soluble extract)	1 gel cap
Kidneys		Probiotics	1 to 5 billion CFU per day. Should include *Enterococcus spp.* Give ¼ to ½ human dose per meal
		Omega-3 fatty acids	300 to 600 milligrams DHA/EPA
		CoQ10	5 to 10 milligrams
		Melatonin	0.3 to 3 milligrams
Heart		Omega-3 fatty acids	300 to 600 milligrams DHA/EPA
		CoQ10	5 to 10 milligrams "Q-Gel" form
		Taurine	250 milligrams
		L-carnitine	250 milligrams
Brain		Omega-3 fatty acids	300 to 600 milligrams DHA/EPA
		CoQ10	5 to 10 milligrams "Q-Gel" form
	Cognitive disorder (senility)	Cholodin (source of choline)	½ tablet for 60 days; or as directed by veterinarian

SYSTEM	CONDITIONS	SUPPLEMENTS	DOSE (Per day unless noted)
Gastro-intestinal system		Digestive enzymes	As directed; or ½ human dose per meal
		Probiotics	1 to 5 billion CFU per day. Should include *Enterococcus spp.* Give ¼ to ½ human dose per meal
		Zypan (pancreas cytosol extract)	¼ tablet per meal
Urinary system	Feline Lower Urinary Tract Disease (FLUTD)	Glucosamine sulfate	250 milligrams
		Mixed antioxidants	⅛ human dose
Skin	Allergies, acne, dry skin, feline hyperesthesia	Omega-3 fatty acids	300 to 600 milligrams DHA/EPA
		Dermatrophin PMG	1 tablet twice a day
Joints	Stiffness, soreness, arthritis	Omega-3 fatty acids	300 to 600 milligrams DHA/EPA
		Hyaluronic acid (Hyalun)	1 to 2 drops
		Glucosamine sulfate	250 milligrams
		MSM	200 milligrams
Respiratory	Upper respiratory; herpes virus	Aeura	Dissolve 1 tablet in 1 ounce (30 ml) water, give 3 to 5 drops twice a day
	Lung disease, asthma	Beta carotene	5 to 10 milligrams per 10 pounds (4.5 kg) body weight
		Probiotics	Should include *Enterococcus* spp. ¼ to ½ human dose per meal
Anti-cancer		Omega-3 fatty acids	2,000 to 5,000 milligrams
		Mixed antioxidants	¼ human dose
		Essiac tea	1 to 2 teaspoons twice a day
		Green tea polyphenol extract (epigallocatechin gallate)	25 milligrams
		Beta-glucans	50 milligrams
		Power Mushrooms	½ tablet twice a day
		Ecklonia cava	½ capsule twice a day
		Chlorophyll (fat-soluble extract)	1 gel cap

Note: When noted that doses should be divided, the total daily dosage should be split into smaller doses and give with meals or as directed. Example: Milk thistle is more effective if small doses are given frequently, so one-quarter of the dose could be given with each of four small meals per day.

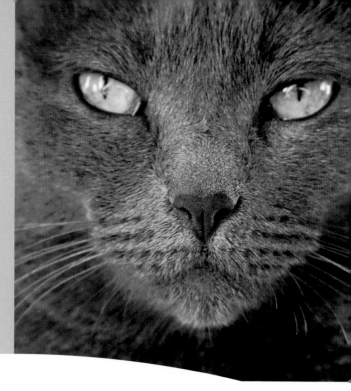

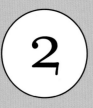

ASTROMEDICINE FOR CATS

Copper-eyed Blue Domestic Shorthair

Why an appendix on astrology in a book about holistic health care for cats? You do not need to use astrology to chart your daily life or that of your cats, but you may be interested in the twelve sun signs of the zodiac and their corresponding personality traits, as they apply to us, our cats, and the special relationship we have with them. Astrology is much more than reading newspaper horoscopes. It can be used as a healing science.

For hundreds of years, we've known that the seasons result from changes in the distance and angle of the sun's rays relative to the Earth, and that the phases of the moon affect the tides, the planting of crops, even the success of the fisherman. It isn't a big leap to suppose these variables affect all living things, including our cats.

The only way we can assist our cats in healing and cleansing their own bodies is to look for clues to appropriate natural remedies or methods of healing. The more aware we become of feline traits and actions, the better equipped we'll be to help our animal companions.

YOUR CAT'S BIRTH SIGN

Beyond what the genetic makeup imparts, the personalities among kittens in a litter tend to be quite similar, even when taking into consideration differences in sex and pecking order. Perhaps this is because they are born close together in time and usually share the same sun sign and several other planetary positions.

Though the serious astrological practitioner would develop a natal horoscope based on the exact time and place of the cat's birth, this isn't absolutely necessary for our purposes. The care, feeding, and spiritual well-being of our cats can benefit enormously if we simply learn about their astrological archetype. If you don't know your cat's birthday or exact age, you could choose a sun sign to celebrate the day you adopted her or the sign closest to her in personality and likeness.

ASTROLOGY AND THE MODERN CAT

Throughout the ages, people have applied astrological principles to every aspect of their physical and spiritual lives. In much the same way, you can explore the twelve sun signs to help you augment your relationship with your cat.

ASTROMEDICINE AND THE SUN SIGNS

Because each of the signs governs a different part of the body, study the information provided for all twelve signs. Earth colors represent the physical plane, and astral colors are ethereal, or more spiritual in nature. As always, consult your holistic practitioner before beginning any treatment.

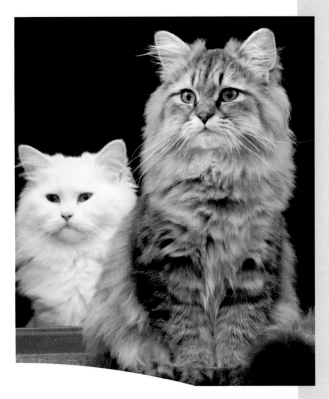

These cats typify Maine Coons or Norwegian Forest Cats, the legendary enchanted cats who appear and disappear at will and see things that we cannot see.

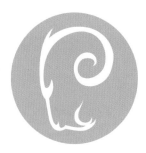

ARIES

(THE RAM)

MARCH 21–APRIL 19

Cardinal element:
FIRE

Ruling planet:
MARS

Earth colors:
CERISE, MAGENTA

Astral colors:
WHITE, ROSE PINK

Gems:
AMETHYST, DIAMOND

Mineral element:
IRON

ARIES, the first sign of the zodiac, represents birth. Aries affects the cerebral nervous system as well as the spinal cord, sensory nerves, pituitary, face, and lower jaw. The planet Mars stimulates the cells, influencing diseases relating to inflammation, fever, and organ lesions. There may be a predisposition to liver problems. An elementary quality of dry heat is associated with this cardinal fire sign.

The Aries cat, in his mind, even when from a large litter, is an only child. Strong and assertive, he makes his needs known when he's hungry. When he wants something, he'll get it. When he's awake, everyone's awake. If he doesn't answer when you call, it's not that he doesn't know his name—the Mars-ruled cat is self-absorbed—he'll get to you when it's convenient for him.

An Aries kitten's charms and naiveté linger into old age. He's cunning and hard to resist. He nearly always gets his own way with people and other animals. He's also fearless and somehow always able to land on his feet. The old motto "If at first you don't succeed" fits him to a T.

As a fire sign, (he shares this element with Leo and Sagittarius), the Aries cat's sunny disposition will cheer you in your darkest hours. Though not usually a lazy cat, the Aries cat does seek warmth and lies in your lap or by your side when you sleep.

The unneutered Aries male is the eternal night stalker and gets into brutal fights, as exemplified by the Greco-Roman god of war, Mars (Ares). Aries can be so aggressive that the chances of his becoming seriously injured or dying in a cat fight are very high. Keep Aries (and all other cats) indoors and spay or neuter them unless they're part of a breeding program. Many of the aggression problems encountered in Aries cats disappear after this procedure. No matter what, they'll never stop believing they're top cat.

The Aries cat is extremely curious and can be accident-prone. He'll love you intensely and share his possessions, but don't try to take something away from him unless it's dangerous, as he will resent you for it. Aries is the sign of authority, after all.

As always, be gentle, as Aries's ego bruises easily. When led with love and given plenty of exercise, this cat will be a champion at everything he does. Whether pedigreed or household pet, the Aries cat is very outgoing and enjoys the spotlight.

To call him extremely intelligent is an understatement. If he could speak in human words, he'd have an answer for everything and would need always to be right. As it is, your life with the Aries cat will be a contest of strength and wit, with never a dull moment.

TAURUS governs the cerebellum, liver, gallbladder, thyroid, throat, and neck, with a possible relationship to kidney problems. The sign of purification, Taurus is ruled by Venus, which controls intercellular fluid and influences infectious diseases. An elementary quality of dry cold is associated with this Earth sign.

The Taurean cat will do whatever she wants whenever she wants. Her shyness is endearing, though it may be frustrating when you'd like to show off her charming ways to friends and neighbors, but she won't perform. Even to animal trainers, the stubborn Taurus proves quite a challenge. However, outside this pigheadedness, Taurus cats are a delight to have underfoot and love to be cuddled on your lap. Taurus cats tend to bond with one person, but they can be magnanimous with their affection.

Taurean people are very outspoken. Without speech, the Taurus cat needs to express herself through physical means, so she needs plenty of exercise. A cat tree made of natural wood and hemp placed next to a sunny window will please her. If you had an aviary or an aquarium, she would delight in watching the birds fly or the tropical fish moving about in the water.

Vibrations and harmony are very important to Taureans' well-being. Harsh or bright light and colors upset them, as do loud noises, so keep the stereo turned low. But they do love sound, such as the jungle, bird, or whale sounds found on nature CD's. Buy one of these, or better yet, make your own recording, reading in your gentlest voice. (Cats of all signs appreciate hearing their human companions' voices.)

Taurus cats have great powers of concentration. They try very hard to understand what you need, but this has to suit them, or the bull emerges victorious. If you're lucky enough to adopt Taurus as a kitten, you'll delight in watching her grow into a magnificent cat.

TAURUS
(THE BULL)
APRIL 20–MAY 20

Cardinal element:
EARTH

Ruling planet:
VENUS

Earth color:
CERISE

Astral colors:
RED, SCARLET, ORANGE, LEMON YELLOW

Gems:
MOSS AGATE, EMERALD

Mineral element:
COPPER

GEMINI

(THE TWINS)

MAY 21–JUNE 21

Cardinal element:
AIR

Ruling planet:
MERCURY

Earth color:
ORANGE

Astral colors:
RED, WHITE, BLUE

Gems:
BERYL, AQUAMARINE, DARK BLUE STONES

Mineral element:
QUICKSILVER (MERCURY)

GEMINI is governed by the planet Mercury. The nervous system, as well as the respiratory system, glands, fibers and tissues, shoulders, paws, and toes are all governed by this sign. An elementary quality of wet heat is associated with Gemini.

Gemini is male and female, extrovert and introvert, aggressive and passive—all rolled into one cat. This animal is a lesson in duality, giving you a full range of emotions and physical attributes. He'll give you a nip asking you to pay attention, then *she*'ll turn around and lick the same spot. He/she, she/he, back and forth. You may think it's typical feline behavior, but no, it's just Gemini.

A Gemini will never be your very own lap cat; this one belongs to the world. When you leave Gemini with the house sitter, you may fret that he'll die without you. But he's happily bonding with the sitter just in case you don't come back, and if you don't, he'll cozy up to the real estate broker, too. It's not that he's fickle; just as the scorpion's nature is to sting, Gemini's is to be all things to all creatures. Just pretend you're as special to him as he makes you feel.

The Gemini cat is a multifaceted, creative cat—poetry in motion. No doubt, he'll create something, even if it's havoc. He's ruled by Mercury, the winged-footed Greek god, so prepare to fly with him as if he were a catbird. However, he can slip through your fingers like quicksilver. Gemini is an air sign and air must circulate freely, so he will want the run of the house.

Gemini won't want to sit still for long though, since he's always in conflict. Just watch that tail swish to and fro. He'll rarely finish anything, including dinner. Instead, he'll be off making mischief somewhere.

Gemini is quick. A bird or mouse doesn't have a chance. He'd like to eat it, but his twin likes to taunt and play with it first—hunger and patience at odds. Could we call him fidgety? No, everyone else is slow. Just let him be, as he changes so fast all his little quirks are here and gone in an instant. His mind sifts through so much so fast that not even the most avid nonverbal communication expert can get it all.

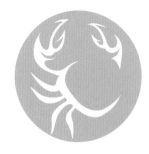

CANCER

(THE CRAB)

JUNE 22–JULY 22

CANCER is ruled by the Moon, which governs cell modularity and the blood. This sign also relates to the breasts, stomach, digestive organs, spleen, and elastic tissues. It is predisposed to diseases of the head and abdomen. Wet cold is the elementary quality associated with this water sign.

The Cancer cat is a gentle creature prone to staring wistfully at you—or at what you may think is nothing—for what seems like an eternity. She's very happy that you keep her inside, as she's most content sitting by the hearth or in any warm, cozy spot.

The Cancer cat's tenacity is unparalleled. Usually the first to arrive at the food bowl and the last to leave it, she'll never let you forget that her sign rules the stomach. Cancer is the most sentimental sign of the zodiac. This means she gets strongly attached to people, animals, and things, so don't reassign a food dish or a bed without her permission.

As a kitten, the Cancer cat will tend to bond with one person. She may run and hide when someone new enters, or stand her ground and hiss if approached. Quite vulnerable, she can be so dedicated to protecting herself that the slightest input can cause her to withdraw. But when left alone at night or separated from her companions, she's likely to cry and moan for the duration.

You may be dismayed when people come to visit and make disparaging remarks about your Cancer cat's moody or unfriendly behavior. It seems only you know that there's a loving creature behind that growl. But if you don't give this cat all the love and security she needs, she may become reclusive. A nonthreatening approach is always best to coax this cat from her shell.

The Cancer cat can change moods quickly and dramatically. Just as the Moon, to us the fastest-moving body in the heavens, may hide behind the clouds and then emerge as a beautiful globe of light in the darkest sky, so does the Cancer cat go through her changes. When she's in touch with the emotional needs of those around her, she can be a great comfort. When she's not in touch, or out of control, she can be miserable.

Cancer cats are motherly. After your female Cancer cat is spayed, and especially if she is the only cat in the family, adopt a kitten for her to nurture. She'll sulk and make a fuss at first, but the bonding that occurs will be profound.

The Cancer cat never forgets anything and is extremely sensitive. Never laugh at her, and be careful not to make her feel foolish. Your Moonchild may get clingy and overbearing sometimes, but she's so endearing that you're likely to love and need her just as much as she needs you.

Cardinal element:
WATER

Ruling planet:
MOON

Earth color:
ORANGE-YELLOW

Astral colors:
GREEN, RUSSET-BROWN

Gems:
PEARL, BLACK ONYX, EMERALD

Mineral element:
SILVER

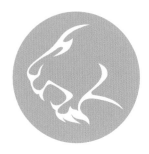

LEO

(THE LION)

JULY 23–AUGUST 22

Cardinal element:
FIRE

Ruling planet:
SUN

Earth colors:
YELLOW, GOLD

Astral colors:
RED, GREEN

Gems:
RUBY, PERIDOT, SARDONYX

Mineral element:
GOLD

LEO governs the heart, circulation, blood, eyes, and vitality. The lion is Leo's symbolic image and is ruled by the Sun. The Sun cat needs to be careful of inflammations. An elementary quality of dry heat is associated with this fire sign.

Leos love to lie in the sun. It's almost impossible to keep them out of it. But be careful because they can burn through those luxurious coats and experience excessive shedding. Seeking warmth to an extreme, they'll lie so close to the fireplace and heat vents that you fear they'll roast.

Leo cats thrive in a positive environment, and they need a tremendous amount of love and admiration. They never seem to get enough lap time or petting, and their appetite for food is hearty. They love to be spoiled, but they give a great deal of love in return. However, it's usually on their terms. If you don't encourage and patronize them a bit, they'll withdraw and brood for a while. This little lion must be given incredible amounts of affection.

Leo cats are very verbal and will have long conversations with you. One meow is seldom enough. They're rarely shy and have a magnificent deep, throaty, purr. They greet people at the door and follow them from room to room.

Always the instigator, Leo marches around your home like the Pied Piper, with everyone following behind. If another cat usurps his position, the lion will most likely stalk off and sulk, awaiting the fond caresses of his "subjects"—you and other members of your household. This little cub plays many roles, including your mother or your baby, depending on whether he's in a giving or a receiving mood. He's sunny by nature and will play with, pounce on, and tease all who enter his kingdom.

Leo usually takes center stage. If you're giving affection to another person or animal, he's sure to get in the middle. I suggest you make a special effort to not let him push another cat away from you, correcting him gently and telling him he'll have his turn. He hates to be scolded or demeaned publicly. Leo doesn't understand the meaning of "wrong" or "bad." He thinks he's always right. However, he does have a great sense of fair play.

Just like Leo people, Leo cats are as theatrical as they are regal. Leo cats need a lot of stimulation, and they love new toys, tiring of old ones quickly. Guard against accidents with Leos, as they often don't think before they leap. They just like to be watched and admired. If your Leo does not fit this profile, he may have had less-than-perfect care during the critical first six weeks of his life.

Be patient and remember to lavish him with praise and affection. You've got a star on your hands, so be prepared to be his fan.

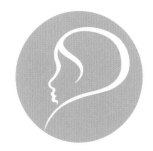

VIRGO

(THE VIRGIN)
AUGUST 23–SEPTEMBER 22

VIRGO is ruled by Mercury, which maintains the nerves. Virgo cats are prone to infections. Virgo governs the bowels, intestines (and everything dependent on them), and solar plexus. This earth sign has an elementary quality of dry cold.

Though quick and alert, Virgos tend to be the most tranquil of all cats, their personality making them the most able to handle unfavorable conditions. Even a Virgo cat has her limits, though, so try not to overload her. She can distress you and then exhibit her own contradictory feline moods, such as wanting to be on your lap but not willing to be held against her will. Win her trust by avoiding the use of force. A Virgo cat is naturally friendly and has a warm disposition, but she can be irritable if you make fun of her. Perceptive and steadfast, she responds best to a gentle approach.

Like the Leo cat, Virgo will usually follow you all over the house as you do chores, content just to see you and be near you. She may be shy with visitors, but with family and regular visitors she won't be at a loss for meows. She tries to communicate with you with sound just as you do with words; listen with your heart as well as your ears.

A Virgo cat is so well mannered and easy to be with, you may tend to favor her. She'll announce herself to feline friends with a polite lick, meaning "May I join you?" If rebuffed, she'll retreat, so always be gentle and sensitive with this beautiful creature. She understands "no" very well and usually doesn't need to be scolded, but if she does, a water squirt bottle does the trick.

The Virgo cat loves routine and dislikes having the furniture moved, let alone her litter box or water bowl, so leave things where they are. However, being a Virgo, she'll adapt to change when necessary. Extremely clean and fastidious, the Virgo cat will groom herself proudly.

A Virgo cat would probably love a friend, but don't buy a breed of cat larger than she is unless you introduce the new arrival as a small kitten. Virgo likes to mother things smaller than herself, and she doesn't want her position to be usurped.

Inquisitive at all times, the Virgo cat must look in every drawer and cupboard, and she hates closed doors. She loves toys and exercise and delights in something new. She loves to have the run of the house to explore.

Virgo cats love to learn, and they often surprise us by mastering new tasks—such as walking on a leash or coming when called—on the first try. However, if you don't help develop Virgo's potential fully, she can become a sad little introvert.

Since a Virgo cat is a good traveler, consider taking her with you when you go on vacation.

Cardinal element:
EARTH

Ruling planet:
MERCURY

Earth color:
CHARTREUSE

Astral colors:
GOLD, BLACK

Gems:
PINK JASPER, SAPPHIRE

Mineral element:
MERCURY

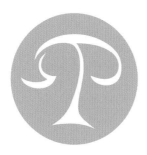

LIBRA

(THE SCALES)

SEPTEMBER 23–OCTOBER 22

Cardinal element:
AIR

Ruling planet:
VENUS

Earth color:
GREEN

Astral colors:
**BLACK, CRIMSON,
LIGHT BLUE**

Gem:
OPAL

LIBRA, ruled by Venus, governs the bladder and kidneys. A cardinal air sign, Libra has an elementary quality of wet heat.

The eternal judge, the Libra cat is part angel, part devil. Usually the peacemaker, he will survey his territory from every conceivable angle. Only then can he make a decision, but Libra defines decisions as something you change your mind about constantly. He loves harmony but remains a paradox himself.

The lesson of this sign is never to give Libra a choice. He hates to make decisions. With his tail always in motion, he's the eternal cat in conflict: "Should I come or should I go?" It's difficult to get him into the groove of a routine, but this is exactly what he needs. Just feed him the same well-balanced fresh foods at the same time in the same place every day; make changes gradually so as not to upset his sense of well-being.

Libra tends to be a bit slow. You call and call him for breakfast, but he's more interested in watching something out the window—a blade of grass or a Saint Bernard. It's not that he's stubborn; he'll come when he wants to.

Don't rush Libra when he's in the litter box. He'll scratch every inch, before and after.

Libras tend to be auditory, and they like music. If you have to leave your Libra cat at home alone, call him often and let him listen to your voice on your answering machine.

Loving and sweet, Libra tends to be a verbal cat who'll purr sweetly, rub up against you, and roll over at your feet. He'll drive you crazy, but you'll end up living to please him and loving every minute.

Your Libra would love to please you, but he'd rather please himself. If you have more than one cat, your Libra will eat from everyone else's plate and snooze in everyone else's bed.

SCORPIO
(THE SCORPION)
OCTOBER 23-NOVEMBER 21

SCORPIO, ruled primarily by Pluto and secondarily by Mars, governs the reproductive organs. Symbolized by the scorpion (and sometimes by the white eagle or the gray lizard), this water sign has an elementary quality of wet cold. Scorpio is ruled by the mythological figure Pluto, lord of the underworld.

The most invincible of signs, a Pluto cat loves a good contest. She'll take on the big guys, even the family dog! Scorpio loves a good fight but, mostly, she likes to win. If Scorpio loses the battle, just wait; she'll be hiding around the corner ready to pounce, and she won't quit until she succeeds.

To maintain a Scorpio cat's sinewy muscles, feed her fresh foods and keep her active. She needs lots of play, but it's not unusual for her to sit by the sidelines watching others make fools of themselves, whether they're cats or humans.

A Scorpio needs firm but loving discipline. Otherwise your Scorpio cat will get what she wants when she wants it! But remember, the Scorpion can sting, so handle her with care and give her lots of love and affection along with your discipline.

If you're blue, your Scorpio cat is likely to be there for you, licking away your tears before anyone else has an inkling that something's wrong. She'll love to share this little secret with you, and you'll be laughing out loud sooner than you think. But don't take it seriously if sometimes she ignores you. She'll be ready to be social again before long.

A Scorpio may be fun and outgoing, but she never forgets anything. She loves to jump or pounce when you least expect it. Afterward, she'll lick your hand, so there's no way you can be angry with her.

The Scorpio cat loves company, but she bonds with one person easily. If you work at home, she'll be content to be with you. If not, she'd like a friend to torment—just a little. Get her a challenging companion; maybe an Aries or a Sagittarius. However, Scorpio cats are fond of the opposite sex, so be sure to spay or neuter them by six months, unless you're planning to use them in a conscientious, responsible breeding program.

Scorpio is a sensuous cat and loves to be groomed. If she's shorthaired, polish her gleaming coat with a chamois. She needs lots of stroking, and she'll rub and nudge you back to thank you.

A Scorpio cat is likely to be a pack rat. If you retrieve your belongings from her cache, leave a little mouse toy in their place. The Scorpio cat may also rediscover a treasured item you thought was gone forever.

Cardinal element:
WATER

Ruling planets:
PLUTO, MARS

Earth color:
BLUE

Astral colors:
GOLDEN, BLACK

Gems:
TOPAZ, MALACHITE

Mineral element:
IRON

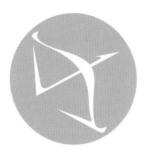

SAGITTARIUS

(THE ARCHER)

NOVEMBER 22–DECEMBER 21

Cardinal element:
FIRE

Ruling planet:
JUPITER

Earth color:
BLUE

Astral colors:
GOLD, RED, GREEN

Gems:
TURQUOISE, DIAMOND

Mineral element:
TIN

SAGITTARIUS is ruled by Jupiter, the planet of expansion, which also affects cell regeneration. This sign relates to the musculature, cardiac system, and blood vessels. A mutable fire sign and the friendliest sign in the zodiac, Sagittarius has an elementary quality of dry heat.

Happy, playful, and clownlike from birth, the Sagittarian cat lives to be loved, petted, and appreciated. The eyes of this little archer are trusting, and he'll be your loving, faithful friend always, especially if you keep him busy learning new things and meeting new people. He's independent, but he'll never deny you your divine right to give him pleasure.

A Sagittarius cat will rarely reject you, your friends, or other pets. He'll cry if you leave him alone. He needs a companion cat from birth, and it's best to adopt a sibling from the same litter, as two Sagittarians are better than one.

Your Sagittarios cat will cuddle in your arms, go for a ride in the car (most love to travel), and may even enjoy cat shows. He'll be happy if you leave an article of your clothing on the floor or in his bed for him to sleep with when you're at work. Better yet, take him with you if you can. But his need for attention is balanced by his desire for freedom. As with all cats, never let him outside, or he may never come back.

The Sagittarian cat may think he's a dog. If you have one, he'll be happy to be friends with it, if you start him young. But if you have a doggie door be careful that your Sagittarian cat doesn't sneak out and call every feline in the neighborhood to come over and play.

Your Sagittarius is forever curious. If this cat could talk, he'd never stop asking you questions. If he knew what hypocrisy meant, he wouldn't stand for it. He may be clumsy, knocking over vases and pulling down tablecloths in his path. Get him a tall scratching post or kitty tree, as he loves to shred things. If he were a person, he'd tear into ideas as enthusiastically as he tears into your couch.

Sagittarius can also be obstinate, and he likes to challenge your authority, especially if he's a big cat. He just doesn't realize how heavy he is when he lands on your stomach and want to cuddle like a kitten. Don't throw him down, just give him the bear hug he seems to crave.

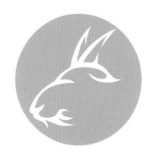

CAPRICORN, ruled by Saturn and represented by the goat, rules the digestive tract and the bones. This sign has an elementary quality of dry cold. It is sometimes ruled by the fish or the unicorn.

Capricorn is an elegant cat, with one of the most intriguing personalities of all the signs. Because of her depth and complexity, she may appear aloof or remote, but this only masks an inherent shyness and introspection.

Capricorn is a feminine sign and forever youthful, but there's something stoic about her even when she's playing. Such intense eyes—when she looks at you, her eyes tell the whole story. Just be receptive to it.

A Capricorn cat is strong-willed and tenacious, with a mind of her own. She doesn't like to be embarrassed and hates to lose. Though she's the most conservative sign in the zodiac, energy is one thing she doesn't conserve. Like the mountain goat, she likes to climb to the highest vantage point and assume dominion over everything and everyone. When it comes to play, she's nonstop and downright silly.

The Capricorn cat will try hard to be a person for you, but remember, she's still a cat. A tidy animal, she'll rarely get dirty or break anything. If she does, she'll be upset, as she wants to be liked and admired.

Watch for hairballs, as Capricorns are meticulous groomers, not only of themselves but of everything else, including you. She loves to let you groom her and bathe her, but if she thinks your guard is down, she'll bolt in a flash. She may sneak outdoors, so be sure she always wears a collar and tag. With patience, you can teach her to walk on a leash. She may skulk, cower, slink, or lie down, but ultimately, she'll enjoy the trip.

A Capricorn cat dreams about birds and anything that will keep her agile body and quick mind moving. She seems to sleep less than most cats, but boredom will knock her right out.

The Capricorn cat matures quickly, but she still wants to be the baby and may be jealous at first of a new addition to the family, so think twice before bringing home a pal. She'd rather have you all to herself for a playmate. But when her supremacy isn't threatened, Capricorn loves other cats, perhaps more than people. And when she challenges a "top cat," she'll end up on top through sheer persistence, and the former ruler won't even realize his position has been usurped.

If you bring home a new friend, be patient. Capricorn will come around eventually, but she'll hiss at the intruder every chance she gets, and she may even ignore you for a while. She's quite serious about her territory and could hurt the new cat. Proceed cautiously. Try changing the subject by giving her catnip or a new toy.

CAPRICORN

(THE GOAT)
DECEMBER 22–JANUARY 19

Cardinal element:
EARTH

Ruling planet:
SATURN

Earth color:
BLUE-VIOLET

Astral colors:
GARNET, SILVER, GRAY, BROWN, BLACK

Gems:
GARNET, WHITE ONYX, MOONSTONE

Mineral element:
LEAD

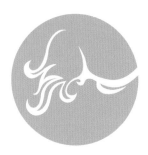

AQUARIUS

(THE WATER CARRIER)

JANUARY 20–FEBRUARY 18

Cardinal element:
AIR

Ruling planets:
URANUS, SATURN

Earth color:
VIOLET

Astral colors:
BLUE, PINK, NILE GREEN

Gems:
AMETHYST, SAPPHIRE, OPAL, TURQUOISE

Mineral element:
ZINC

AQUARIUS is ruled by Uranus. Aquarius is an air sign, with an elementary quality of wet heat. This sign governs the legs, ankles, circulatory system, and blood.

Aquarius is strong, trusting, fearless, and courageous, but also sensitive. The Aquarian cat is incredibly psychic: he seems to know without knowing how he knows. There is nothing average about Aquarius. He's the most precocious cat in the house, and becomes top cat before you know it. He loves freedom and is very independent.

Male or female, Aquarian cats will talk to you incessantly. Most love people and tolerate other pets nicely, but they know you love them best and share that secret with you. They'll ignore you sometimes when you call, but they come running when they're ready (just a few moments later than you'd like). They're unpredictable and contradictory—one moment calm and docile and suddenly wound up like a tornado.

Great eaters as well as very good athletes, Aquarian cats love to climb as high as they can and dive-bomb from the top of the shutters, drapes, or cat trees. They'll jump into the air and expect you to catch them. They'll ride on your shoulders like a scarf. They do somersaults and roll over on their backs, sometimes falling asleep in that position, a hilarious sight.

With this perpetual clown, you'll never know what to expect. He can become best friends with a dog, a pot-bellied pig, even a horse or a goat! He's so outgoing and fearless that these other creatures just accept him as one of their own. Aquarius has a capacity to love beyond that of any other sign in the zodiac.

PISCES, the twelfth and last sign of the zodiac, is ruled by Neptune and Jupiter and represents change and the consciousness of the soul. This sign governs the arterial blood, red corpuscles, and feet. Cats born under this sign may be susceptible to diseases of the chest. Pisces is a water sign, with an elementary quality of wet cold.

Sweet, gentle, endearing, and magical—part elf, part leprechaun—a Pisces cat grabs at your heartstrings, and before you know it, you're the proud adoptive parent of a Pisces cat.

Pisces are truly sensitive creatures. They see, hear, and smell many things, such as spirits, that we might not know are there.

Pisceans are the keepers of thousands of years of secrets. Tune into them, and you'll be amazed at what they'll tell you.

The Pisces cat needs to remain still for periods of time, otherwise, she's pulled in opposing directions, constantly in conflict. Her sign is symbolized by two fishes: one swimming toward the source of the water and the other toward the sea.

A Pisces's tendency to be dreamy makes it easy for her to leave her body. Your Pisces cat may learn this technique early in life to avoid reprimands. She simply tunes out, traveling to realms of safety on the wings of fantasy. Give her lots of attention and encourage her to be outgoing because if you don't she'll be shy forever. But respect her privacy when she's in a mysterious mood, and let her be.

Pisces loves to love, but they get stressed easily. Your Pisces cat seems perfect, although you might be letting her get away with a lot. She'll charm you into getting her own way, so you may as well surrender. But she'll never abuse you for this or let you spoil her too much; she's too loving for that. Because she makes up her own rules, you must gently let her know what yours are. Use positive reinforcement and avoid the negative.

Pisces cats have their own schedules. They'll sleep when they want to, eat when they want to, and play when they want to, so you may just have to adjust your schedule to theirs.

It's important to protect a Pisces cat from bullies, animal or human, as she doesn't understand and can't tolerate aggression or violence. The music of Chopin or Mozart (both Pisceans) will soothe her.

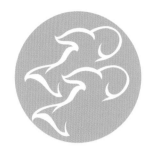

PISCES

(THE FISH)
FEBRUARY 19–MARCH 20

Cardinal element:
WATER

Ruling planets:
NEPTUNE, JUPITER

Earth colors:
CERISE, MAGENTA

Astral colors:
**WHITE, PINK,
EMERALD GREEN, BLACK**

Gems:
**CHRYSOLITE, PINK SHELL,
MOONSTONE**

Mineral element:
TIN

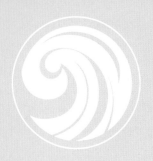

GLOSSARY

ACUPUNCTURE: A holistic therapy that stimulates certain points along various meridians. There are several methods of acupuncture used on cats in holistic veterinary medicine such as aquapuncture, electrostimulation, and laser.

ADJUVANTS: Substances used in vaccines that stimulate inflammation and increase the immune response. An adjuvanted vaccine usually contains a killed virus or organism.

ALLOPATHIC: Pertaining to conventional medicine, also commonly referred to as Western medicine.

ANTIAGING: Preventing or delaying degenerative changes associated with advancing age.

ANTIBODIES: Blood proteins manufactured by immune system B-lymphocytes that attack and destroy invading organisms; antibody production is the goal of vaccination.

ANTIOXIDANT: A substance that destroys oxygen free radicals.

AROMATHERAPY: The use of scent from essential oils to treat mental and physical conditions.

ASTROMEDICINE: A branch of astrology which studies tendencies of a person or animal toward health and sickness, indicating the periods in which they are most vulnerable to disease.

AURA: A colorful energetic "halo" all around the body. Also called the etheric double.

AUTOANTIBODIES: Antibodies that react against the body's own tissues.

AUTOIMMUNE: Referring to a condition in which antibodies react to and destroy the body's own tissues. Examples include lupus, canine hypothyroidism, and immune-mediated hemolytic anemia.

AUTOLOGOUS: "Self-grown"; derived from or transformed to the same individual body.

AYURVEDIC MEDICINE: From the Sanskrit "āyus" (life), and "veda" (science), Ayurveda is a 5,000-year-old system of medicine developed in ancient India that strives to balance the three doshas (and maintain health) within the individual through lifestyle and diet.

B-LYMPHOCYTES: White blood cells that are part of the immune system; when stimulated, they produce antibodies.

BIOAVAILABILITY: The degree to which a food or other substance is digested, absorbed into the bloodstream, and can be or is used by the body.

BIOPHOTONS: The faint light emitted by all living cells; potential uses include diagnostics (sick cells emit more light) and treatment.

BIORESONANCE: The quality of harmony between two living beings. In holistic healing, the term is used to describe a multitude of techniques and devices used to diagnose and/or treat illnesses through energy fields.

CHAKRA: One of the seven main energetic centers of the body.

CHIROPRACTIC: A hands-on healing technique that seeks to correct subluxations, which are small misalignments between vertebrae.

COLOSTRUM: A thin yellowish fluid secreted by the mammary glands of mammals at the time of parturition that is rich in antibodies and minerals and precedes the production of true milk. Also called first milk.

CONSTITUTIONAL HOMEOPATHY: Homeopathic practitioners can select remedies for their patients based upon a constitutional type of prescribing. They select remedies that match descriptions defined in homeopathic repertories as closely as possible and gives only one remedy at a time. Also called classical homeopathy.

CURE: The only goal of homeopathy meaning that the body eliminates the whole disease, not just symptoms, and rises to a state of optimum health.

DENATURE: To distort or alter the fundamental nature of a substance; for instance, to denature a protein means that it loses its natural shape. Denatured proteins are thought to be more allergenic than normal proteins.

DETOXIFICATION: For our purposes, a natural phase of the healing process that occurs as changes in your cat's diet and environment are made. These changes remove the residue and effects of drugs, vaccines, anesthesia, chemicals, processed pet food, and infectious agents. During detoxification, things may seem to get worse for a time, even though the body is actually moving forward to restore health and balance.

DOSHA: In Ayurvedic medicine, there are five elements defined as earth, water, fire, air, and ether. These elements are then organized into three main principals (doshas) in the body, and each individual contains a unique collage of these three basic doshas: vata (air/wind), pitta (fire/sun), and kapha (earth/water).

ELECTROMAGNETIC FIELDS (EMFS): All plants and animals operate by tiny electrochemical pulses at about the same frequency as the energy field on the Earth. Cell phones, computers, televisions, and other appliances all produce toxic EMFs.

EPIGENETICS: Refers to the stable and heritable changes in gene expression that are not attributable to the DNA sequence. The field of epigenetics studies the molecular mechanism by which the environment controls gene activity.

EUTHANASIA: Literally, "good death;" used to describe the humane killing of an animal. In pets, this is typically done through injection of an overdose of barbiturates.

FELDENKREIS METHOD: A therapeutic touch technique that opens new neurological pathways to the brain through the use of nonhabitual movements.

FELINE LOWER URINARY TRACT DISEASE (FLUTD): A catch-all term used to describe a variety of bladder conditions in cats, including idiopathic interstitial cystitis (similar to bladder infections in women), crystals, stones, and blockages.

FEVER: A body temperature above 102°F (38.9°C). A fever can be caused by stress, infection, immune system dysfunction such as an autoimmune disease, or cancer.

FLOWER ESSENCE: A specially prepared energetic extract of flowers and other substances. They act as gentle catalysts to alleviate underlying causes of stress and restore emotional balance.

HABITUAL HOLDING PATTERN: Living things develop compensatory patterns, or ways of holding and defending against a variety of physical and emotional insults. These holding patterns form cellular memory, which is a memory experienced in the tissue at a cellular level.

HEALTH: Not just the absence of symptoms, but an overall feeling of well being and vitality.

HEPATIC: Related to the liver.

HOLISTIC: A philosophy of well-being that considers the physical, mental, emotional, and spiritual aspects of life as closely interconnected and balanced. A holistic approach to veterinary medicine takes into account the breed, lifestyle, diet, activity level, and social environment of a cat as well as the medical history and current symptoms.

HIMALAYAN SALT LAMP: A decorative lamp (not a candle) made from mined Himalayan salt, which is said to naturally produce negative ions that the heat of the lamp release into the ambient environment; helps to combat the effects of EMFs.

HOMEOPATHY: A system of healing developed by Dr. Samuel Hahnemann, a German medical doctor, in the late eighteenth century. The principles of homeopathy include the Law of Similars and the Minimum Dose.

INOCULATION: To physically introduce or inject a microorganism, such as with a vaccine, or a friendly bacteria taken into the gastrointestinal tract, as in probiotic therapy.

MERIDIANS: A system of interconnected pathways through which flows the energy (qi) of the body. Hundreds of acupuncture points, which are also known as acupoints, occur along these pathways.

NANOTECHNOLOGY: The study of control of matter on an atomic or molecular scale. A nanometer (nm) is one billionth of a meter; a strand of DNA is about 2 nm across. Nanotechnology has many intriging potential uses in medicine.

NEGATIVE IONS: Negatively charged particles that are experienced during rain, at the sea shore, near a waterfall, or in a forest.

NEUTER: Surgical sterilization; removal of the male reproductive glands (testes). Also referred to as de-sexing and altering.

NOSODES: Homeopathically prepared remedies made from disease material, such as tissues, discharges, or secretions. They can be used to treat infectious diseases and are sometimes used as a part of a prevention protocol in much the same way vaccines are used.

NUTRACEUTICALS: Nutritional supplementation for a specific purpose, such as glucosamine and MSM for arthritis.

OBLIGATE CARNIVORE: An animal obliged to eat meat, such as the cat, whose strict nutritional requirements are met through its species-specific diet, raw prey.

OPERANT CONDITIONING: A stimulus-response behavior modification (training) method for cats based on the way all animals learn.

OXIDATION: In the body, the process of using oxygen to create energy. This process occurs in the mitochondria, which are small organs also known as organelles within each cell.

PALLIATION: To alleviate symptoms; such as how aspirin treats pain.

PATHOGEN: Any disease-causing organism.

PATHOLOGICAL: Abnormal, unhealthy, causing or contributing to disease.

POSITIVE IONS: Positively charged particles that are found more in desert habitats and where there is a lot of concrete.

QI: From Traditional Chinese Medicine, the vital life force present in all living beings. Also known as chi or energy.

RADIONICS: A bioresonance therapy that purportedly creates healing on an energetic level. Radionics uses a specially designed electronic instrument to diagnose illness and broadcast healing frequencies across a distance.

REIKI: A system of hands-on energy healing developed in Japan from techniques used in ancient Asian cultures.

RENAL: Pertaining to the kidneys.

SPAY: Surgical sterilization; removal of the female reproductive organs (ovaries and uterus) of the female cat; technically called ovariohysterectomy. Also called de-sexing.

SPECIES-SPECIFIC DIET: The diet an animal would eat in its natural habitat.

SUBLUXATION: Small misalignments between vertebrae that are the focus of chiropractic treatment. A luxation is a complete dislocation.

SUCCUSSION: In homeopathy, the violent shaking or pounding of a vial of liquid remedy to increase its therapeutic power. Originally, succussion was the pounding of the diluted remedy against the heel of the hand. Today, homeopathic pharmacies today make remedies by machine.

SUPPRESSION: This term in homeopathy is used to explain how we can get rid of specific symptoms, but it drives the disease into other channels by denying the body's expression of the original disease. Suppressive medicines are often named "anti," such as antibiotics, antipyretics, and anti-inflammatories.

TONKINESE CAT: A pedigreed cat originally created by crossing the Siamese cat with the Burmese cat.

VACCINATION: Inoculation with a vaccine to induce an immunological response to a particular disease.

VACCINOSIS: In homeopathic medicine, a chronic condition with multiple symptoms caused by vaccinations.

VERTEBRAE: One segment of the vertebral column, which is also called the spine or backbone.

VETERINARY ORTHOPEDIC MANIPULATION (VOM): A hands-on healing technology that locates areas of the animal's nervous system that have fallen out of communication and re-establishes neuronal communication.

The Rainbow Bridge

Just this side of heaven is a place called the Rainbow Bridge.

When an animal dies that has been especially close to someone here, that pet goes to the Rainbow Bridge. There are meadows and hills for all of our special friends so they can run and play together. There is plenty of food, water, and sunshine, and our friends are warm and comfortable.

All the animals who had been ill and old are restored to health and vigor. Those who were hurt or maimed are made whole and strong again, just as we remember them in our dreams of days and times gone by. The animals are happy and content, except for one small thing; they each miss someone very special to them who had to be left behind.

They all run and play together, but the day comes when one suddenly stops and looks into the distance. His bright eyes are intent. His eager body quivers. Suddenly he begins to run from the group, flying over the green grass, his legs carrying him faster and faster.

You have been spotted, and when you and your special friend finally meet, you cling together in joyous reunion, never to be parted again. The happy kisses rain upon your face; your hands again caress the beloved head, and you look once more into the trusting eyes of your pet, so long gone from your life but never absent from your heart.

Then you cross the Rainbow Bridge together.

—Author Unknown

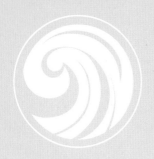

RESOURCES

BOOKS

AROMATHERAPY, FLOWER ESSENCES, AND HERBS

Grosjean, Nelly. *Veterinary Aromatherapy.* Saffron Walden, UK: C. W. Daniel Co, 2005. www.nellygrosjean.com

Hofve, Jean, D.V.M. *Bach Flower Remedies for Cats.* Boulder, CO: Little Big Cat, Inc., 2006. www.littlebigcat.com

Wulff-Tilford, Mary, and Gregory Tilford. *All You Ever Wanted to Know About Herbs for Pets.* Irvine, CA: BowTie Press, 2001.

BEHAVIOR AND TRAINING

Fields-Barbineau, Miriam. *Cat Training in 10 Minutes.* Neptune City, NJ: TFH Publications, 2003. www.miriamfields.com

Pryor, Karen. *Getting Started: Clicker Training For Cats.* Waltham, PA: Sunshine Books, 2003. www.clickertraining.com

HANDS-ON HEALING

Fox, Michael W., BVet.Med., Ph.D., D.Sc. *The Healing Touch: The Proven Massage Program for Cats. Revised edition.* New York: Newmarket Press, 2004. www.doctormwfox.org

Fulton, Elizabeth, and Kathleen Prasad. *Animal Reiki.* Berkeley, CA: Ulysses Press, 2006. www.animalreikisource.com

Tellington-Jones, Linda. *Getting in TTouch with Your Cat: A New and Gentle Way to Harmony, Behavior and Well-Being.* North Pomfret, VT: Trafalgar Square Press, 2003. www.ttouch.com

Zidonis, Nancy A., and Amy Snow. *Acu-Cat: A Guide to Feline Acupressure.* Denver, CO: Tall Grass Publications, 2000. www.animalacupressure.com

HOLISTIC AND HOMEOPATHIC CARE

Arora, Sandy. *Whole Health for Happy Cats: A Guide to Keeping your Cat Naturally Healthy, Happy, and Well-Fed.* Quarry Books, 2006.

Chambreau, Christina, D.V.M. *Healthy Animal's Journal: What You Can Do to Have Your Dog or Cat Live a Long and Healthy Life.* Sparks, NV: TRO Productions, 2003. www.christinachambreau.com

Hamilton, Don, D.V.M. *Homeopathic Care for Cats and Dogs: Small Doses for Small Animals.* Berkeley, CA: North Atlantic Books, 1999.

Pottenger, Francis M. *Pottenger's Cats: A Study In Nutrition.* La Mesa, CA: Price-Pottenger Foundation, 2005. www.ppnf.org

Yarnall, Celeste, Ph.D. *Natural Cat Care: A Complete Guide to Holistic Health Care for Cats.* Edison, NJ: Castle, 2000. www.celestialpets.com

Yarnall, Celeste, Ph.D. *Natural Dog Care: A Complete Guide to Holistic Health Care for Dogs.* Edison, NJ: Castle, 2000. www.celestialpets.com

Zucker, Martin. *Veterinarians' Guide to Natural Remedies for Cats: Safe and Effective Alternative Treatments and Healing Techniques from the Nations' Top Holistic Veterinarians.* New York: Three Rivers Press, 2000.

IMMUNIZATION AND VACCINES

Coulter, Harris L., and Barbara Loe Fisher. *A Shot in the Dark.* New York: Avery Publishing, 1991.

O'Driscoll, Catherine. *What Vets Don't Tell You About Vaccines.* England: Abbeyville Press, 1998.

NEW AGE, QUANTUM HEALING, AND ANTIAGING

Ebertin, Reinhold. *Astrological Healing: The History and Practice of Astromedicine.* York Beach, ME: Samuel Weiser Inc., 1990.

Emoto, Masaru. *The Hidden Messages in Water.* Hillsboro, OR: Beyond Words Publ., 2001. www.masaru-emoto.net

Lipton, Bruce H, Ph.D. *The Biology of Belief, Unleashing the Power of Consciousness, Matter and Miracles.* Santa Rosa, CA: Mountain Love /Elite Books, 2005.

McTaggart, Lynne. *The Field, the Quest for the Secret Force of the Universe.* New York: Harper Books, 2008.

Melody. A. *Love is in the Earth: A Kaleidoscope of Crystals— The Reference Book Describing Metaphysical Properties of the Mineral Kingdom (Update).* Richland, WA: Earth-Love Publishing House, Limited, 1995.

Perry, Wayne. *Sound Medicine: The Complete Guide to Healing with the Human Voice.* Franklin Lakes, NJ: New Page Books, 2007. www.wayneperry.com

Talbot, Michael. *The Holographic Universe.* New York: HarperCollins, 1992.

Wiley, T. S., and Julie Taguchi, M.D. *Sex, Lies, and Menopause.* New York: HarperCollins, 2000. www.thewileyprotocol.com

Wiley, T .S., with Bent Formby, Ph.D. *Lights Out: Sugar, Sleep, and Survival.* New York: Simon & Schuster, 2000. www.thewileyprotocol.com

NONVERBAL COMMUNICATION

Blake, Stephen, D.V.M. *The Pet Whisperer: Stories about My Friends, the Animals.* San Diego, CA: The Pet Whisperer Publ., 2003. www.thepetwhisperer.com

Milani, Myrna, D.V.M. *The Body Language and Emotion of Cats: What Your Cat is Trying To Tell You.* New York: Morrow, 1987. www.mmilani.com

Schoen, Allen M. *Kindred Spirits.* New York: Broadway, 2001. www.drschoen.com

Smith, Penelope. *Animal Talk: Interspecies Telepathic Communication.* Hillsboro, OR: Beyond Words Publishing, 2008. www.animaltalk.net

PEST CONTROL

Olkowski, William, Sheila Dear, and Helga Olkowski. *Common Sense Pest Control: Least Toxic Solutions for Your Home, Garden, Pets and Community.* Newtown, CT: Taunton Press, 1991.

Sammons, Chip. *Flea Control: A Holistic and Humorous Approach.* Clackamas, OR: Holistic Pet Center, 1996.

PET LOSS

Congalton, David, and Charlotte Alexander. *When Your Pet Outlives You: Protecting Animal Companions After You Die.* Troutdale, OR: New Sage Press, 2002.

Nieburg, Herbert, and Arlene Fisher. *Pet Loss: A Thoughtful Guide for Adults and Children.* New York: Harper Paper Backs, 1996.

Sheridan, Kim. *Animals and the Afterlife: True Stories of Our Best Friends' Journey Beyond Death.* Carlsbad, CA: Hay House, 2006. www.animalsandtheafterlife.com www.kimsheridan.com

Smith, Penelope. *Animals in Spirit.* Hillsboro, OR: Beyond Words Publishing, 2008. www.animaltalk.net

SUPPLIERS

CAT LITTER

GPC Pet Products
877.367.9225
www.worldsbestcatlitter.com
Manufacturer/distributor of World's Best Cat Litter

West Oregon Wood Products, Inc.
503.397.6707
www.wowpellets.com
Manufacturer of Noah's Choice Premium Animal Bedding

ENCLOSURES AND CARRIERS

Cat Fence-In Kits
888.738.9099
www.catfencein.com

Sherpa Pet Group
800.743.7723
www.sherpapet.com

SturdiProducts, Inc.
800.779.8193
www.sturdiproducts.com

FLOWER ESSENCES

Flower Essence Services
www.fesflowers.com

Spirit Essences Holistic Remedies for Animals
877.857.7474
www.spiritessence.com
Founded by Jean Hofve, D.V.M., in 1995, Spirit Essences remains the only line of essence remedies formulated by a veterinarian.

FULL-SPECTRUM LIGHTING

Duro-Test Lighting Corp.
800.289.3876
www.durotest.com

Full Spectrum Solutions, Inc.
888.574.7014
www.fullspectrumsolutions.com

HOMEOPATHIC RESOURCES

Aeura, Inc.
800.430.6747
www.aeura.com

Capitol Drugs
800.819.9098
www.capitoldrugs.com

GUNA, Inc.
888.486.2835
www.gunainc.com

Heel, Inc. (for practitioners) Heel/BHI
800.621.7644
www.heelusa.com

Natural Health Supplies
888.689.1608
www.a2zhomeopathy.com

Similasan Homeopathic Remedies
800.426.1644
www.similasanusa.com
Homeopathic eye drops

MISCELLANEOUS PRODUCTS

Aromatherapy Hydrosol Mists
www.celestialpets.com

Corning Inc. World Kitchen LLC
800.999.3436
www.pyrexware.com
*Pyrex glass bowls with airtight lids
for fresh, raw food storage*

Eng3 Corporation
877.571.9206
 www.eng3corp.com
Manufacturers and distributors of the Activated Air device

Feel-Rite Pet Products, Inc.
866.928.9007
www.magnamat.com
*Manufacturers of the Magna-Mat line of magnetic/orthopedic
pet beds, pads, and mats*

Himalayan Pure Crystal Salt Products
www.celestialpets.com
Lamps, candle holders, bath salts, and table salt

Lyon Technologies, Inc.
888.LYON.USA
www.lyonusa.com
Distributors of Thermotex infra-red heating pads and pet beds

Ojibwa Tea of Life
www.ojibwatea.com
*Essiac tea and other herbal products, all 100 percent
organic and ethically wildcrafted*

Purple Plates
www.purpleplates.com
Tesla's purple positive energy plates, disks, and pet collars

Vet Serv 800.421.0026
www.vetserv-usa.com
Veterinary supply company

YUK 2e Vet Planet
www.vetplanet.net
*A safe, nontoxic, but terrible tasting gel to deter pets from licking
wounds, lesions, splints, and IV catheters*

MUSIC

Music for Pets and People
860.567.9217
www.musicforpetsandpeople.com

NONTOXIC CLEANING AND PEST CONTROL

Fleabusters, Inc.
800.666.3532
www.fleabusters.com
*Flea treatment; dust mite and yard products
(beneficial nematodes) are also available*

Pure Comfort Shampoos
www.celestialpets.com
*Erigeron canadensis (Canadian Fleabane) shampoo
and other products*

Seventh Generation
800.456.1191
www.seventhgeneration.com
*Green cleaning and laundry products, paper goods, baby and
feminine products. Free e-newsletter and coupons available.*

PET LOSS

Cal Pet Crematory, Inc.
818.983.2313
www.calpet.com
*The cat's remains can be shipped frozen using overnight mail.
Extremely reliable group that insures you get your cats ashes
back.*

SUPPLEMENTS AND WHOLE FOOD PRODUCTS

Celestial Pets Natural Nutrition & Holistic Health Care
818.707.6331
www.celestialpets.com

*Supplier of the essentials to make your own homemade pet diet,
including Celestial Cats Vitamin Mineral Plus Feline Supplement,
Celestial Cats Essential Fatty Acid Oil blend, Celestial Cats Feline
Enzyme Supplement, and Celeste Yarnall Foods (flash-frozen,
naturally-raised human grade meat and poultry)*

See website for a complete list of available supplements, and/or call for information regarding clinical nutrition services and products mentioned throughout this book.

Celestial Pets also distributes colostrum product, grapefruit seed extract, omega-3 fatty acids and essential fatty acid blends, salba, and clustered water solutions.

Hyalun Oral Hyaluronic Acid (HA)
866.318.8484
www.hyalun.com
Hyaluronic acid supplement

MVP Laboratories, Inc.
800.856.4648
www.mvplabs.com
Cholodin, choline-loading dietary supplements

Nutramax Laboratories
888.886.6442
www.nutramaxlabs.com
Liver support products

Only Natural Pet
888.937.6677
www.onlynaturalpet.com
"Immune Strengthener," a blend of natural vitamins, herbs, antioxidants, and medicinal mushrooms

Optimum Choices
866.305.2306
www.optimumchoices.com
Blue-green algae products for pets and people

Pet's Friend
800.868.1009
www.mypetsfriend.com
Dr. Russell Swift's enzyme formulas, multiple glandular and organ concentrates, feline enzyme supplements, trace minerals, and other natural healing products including Celestial Cats VM+ and Celestial Cats feline enzyme supplements

Probiotic Clinical Nutrition Protocol By Celestial Pets Clinical Nutrition Services Probiotic supplement not destroyed by stomach acids Available by consultation only. (See Celeste Yarnall, Ph.D., under "Professional Specialists")

VISUAL MEDIA

Applied Kinesiology
Free video available on the Internet explaining Applied Kinesiology and Muscle Testing: "Applied Kinesiology Muscle Testing Food Products"
www.youtube.com/watch?v=2q9JTWEz8Fc

Giving a Cat Subcutaneous Fluids
Free video available on the Internet: www.hubpages.com/hub/Giving-a-cat-subcutaneous-fluids

WATER RESOURCES

Multi-Pure Drinking Water Systems
800.622.9206
www.multipureco.com
Water filtration systems

Quantum Age Water Stirwands
www.quantumagewater.com
Water balancing system

Willard Water CAW Industries, Inc.
www.dr-willardswater.com
Catalyst Altered Water (CAW)

VETERINARY PRACTITIONERS

Susan Beal, D.V.M.
Big Run Healing Arts
Big Run, PA 15715 814.427.5004
Veterinary specialist in homeopathy, cranial sacral therapy, and veterinary chiropractic. Available for telephone consultation

Bert H. Brooks, D.V.M. Melissa Brooks, B.S.
Cache Creek Vet Service
Woodland, CA
530.666.7322
www.cchvs.com
*NAET, ETA, Harmonic Translation
Available for telephone consultation*

Christina Chambreau, D.V.M.
Sparks, MD
410.771.4968
www.christinachambreau.com
www.healthyanimalsjournal.com
Member of the Academy of Veterinary Homeopathy. Courses given on veterinary homeopathy. Available for telephone consultation.

W. Jean Dodds, D.V.M.
Santa Monica, CA
310.828.4804
www.hemopet.org
Founder and president of Hemopet

Michael W. Lemmon, D.V.M.
Renton, WA
425.226.8418

Charles E. Loops, D.V.M.
Pittsboro, NC
919.542.0442
www.charlesloopsdvm.com
Available for telephone consultation regarding homeopathy, nosodes, and vaccination issues

Richard Pitcairn, D.V.M., Ph.D.
Animal Natural Health Center
www.drpitcairn.com
Teacher and lecturer on homeopathy and nutrition, and post graduate instruction for veterinarians

Russell Swift, D.V.M.
Tamarac, FL
877.BE.WELL 2
www.therightremedy.com
Classical homeopath and veterinary chiropractor. Available for telephone consultation

PROFESSIONAL SPECIALISTS

Gary Craig Emotional Freedom Technique (EFT)
www.emofree.com

Laurel Denham
805.570.9666
Animal psychic. Available for telephone consultations

Tapas Fleming TAT Life
877.674.4344
www.tatlife.com
Creator of the Tapas Acupressure Technique

Carol Gurney
818.597.1154
www.animalcommunicator.net
Animal communicator and bodywork

Lydia Hiby
760.796.4304
www.lydiahiby.com
Animal communicator/analyst and author

William L. Inman, B.S., D.V.M., CVCP
208.772.4360
www.vomtech.com
Teacher and lecturer, developed the Veterinary Orthopedic Manipulation (VOM) technique

Laura Mignosa, NCCH
860.666.5064
www.ctherbschool.com
Nationally certified Chinese herbalist

Wayne Perry
800.276.8634
www.wayneperry.com
Founder and director of the Sound Therapy Center of Los Angeles

Kathleen Prasad
415.420.9783
www.animalreikisource.com
Reiki master

Joan R. Ranquet
888.882.7208
www.joanranquet.com
Animal communicator, author, and teacher

Michael H. Scholes
310.827.7737
www.labofflowers.com
Aromatherapy consultant; aromatic supplies and hydrosols

Kate Solisti
303.568.9048
www.akinshipwithanimals.com
Animal communicator and author, classes and one-on-one mentoring/apprenticeships, nutritional consultations

Linda Tellington-Jones
866.488.6824
www.ttouch.com
Founder and instructor of the Tellington TTouch method. Books, videos, and training available

Patty Smith-Verspoor, DMH, DVH, HD (RHom.), BSEd
Doctor of Veterinary Heilkunst
613.692.6950 (clinic)
www.homeopathy.com/clinic
www.heilkunst.com

Marla S. Wilson
805.426.9647
www.marlasapothecary.com
www.abbp.org
Aromatherapist, aromatherapy instructor, and anthroposophic orgonomic therapist

Celeste Yarnall, Ph.D.
818.707.6331
www.celestialpets.com
Available for consultations regarding the fresh/raw food diet and supplementation and alternative healing therapies for cats and dogs

ASSOCIATIONS, ORGANIZATIONS, AND SERVICES

The Association for BioResonance and BioFeedback Practitioners
www.abbp.org

Academy of Veterinary Homeopathy
www.theavh.org

AltVetMed: Complementary and Alternative Veterinary Medicine
www.altvetmed.org

The American Academy of Veterinary Acupuncture
www.aava.org

American Association of Cat Enthusiasts
www.aaceinc.org

American Cat Fanciers' Association
www.acfacat.com

American Holistic Veterinary Medical Association
www.ahvma.org
Publishes the Journal of the American Holistic Veterinary Medical Association *practitioner directory*
www.holisticvetlist.com

American Institute of Homeopathy
www.homeopathyusa.org
Publishes the Journal of the American Institute of Homeopathy

Animal Poison Control Center (USA)
Animal poison-related emergency information, twenty-four-hours/seven days a week

American Veterinary Chiropractic Association
www.animalchiropractic.org

Association of British Veterinary Acupuncturists
www.abva.co.uk

Association of Veterinary Acupuncturists of Canada
www.avac.ca

Association Scientific Italian Acupuncture Veterinary sans Frontiere
www.scuoladiagopuntura.it

Australian Veterinary Chiropractic Association
www.chirovet.com.au

Bio-Integral Resource Center
510.524.2567
www.birc.org

British Association of Holistic Nutrition and Medicine
www.bahnm.org.uk

British Association of Homeopathic Veterinary Surgeons
www.bahvs.com

Canadian Cat Association
www.cca-afc.com

Cat Fanciers' Association
www.cfainc.org
Publishers of the Cat Fanciers' Almanac

CHI Institute
www.tcvm.com

Energetic Medicine Research
www.energetic-medicine.net (info)
www.energetic-healing.com (store)

Flower Essence Society
www.flowersociety.org

German Veterinary Acupuncture Society
www.gervas.org

Governing Council of the Cat Fancy
www.gccfcats.org

Grief Recovery Institute
www.grief-recovery.com

Holistic Health for Animals Association
828.369.8711

International Cat Agility Training
www.catagility.com

The International Cat Association
www.tica.org

International Foundation for Nutrition and Health
www.ifnh.org

International Veterinary Acupuncture Directory
www.komvet.at

International Veterinary Acupuncture Society
www.ivas.org

NAET practitioners www.holisticvetlist.com
www.naet.com

National Animal Supplement Council
www.nasc.cc
Nonprofit industry group dedicated to protecting and enhancing the health of companion animals and horses; certifies products meeting its rigorous standards

National United Professional Association of Trained Homeopaths (Canada)
www.nupath.org

Natural Rearing Breeders Directory
www.nrbreeders.homestead.com

New Zealand Holistic Animal Therapists Association
www.nzhata.org.nz

Novalis Organon
www.novalisorganon.com
Alternative medical school curriculum based on Anthroposophic Orgonomy

The Pacific Institute of Aromatherapy
www.pacificinstituteofaromatherapy.com

Price-Pottenger Nutrition Foundation
www.ppnf.org

Veterinary Acupuncture Association (the Netherlands)
www.snva.nl

Veterinary Advice Line
www.vetadviceline.com

Veterinary Botanical Medical Association
www.vbma.org

Veterinary Institute of Integrative Medicine
www.viim.org

Washington Animal Disease Diagnostic Lab
509.335.9696
Provides necropsy services

Weston A. Price Foundation
www.westonaprice.org

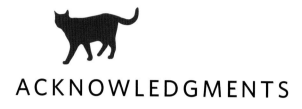

ACKNOWLEDGMENTS

FOR THEIR INVALUABLE CONTRIBUTIONS TO THIS PROJECT, I WOULD LIKE TO THANK THE FOLLOWING PEOPLE.

My devoted friend and Celestial Pets business partner, Imelda Lopez-Casper, for her invaluable assistance in the preparation of this book.

Jean Hofve, D.V.M., for all her help and contributions. Collaborating with Jean has been a pleasure, and I am grateful to this dear friend for sharing her veterinary knowledge and experience.

Russell Swift, D.V.M., of Pets Friend, for sharing his expertise through the years.

Christina Chambreau, D.V.M., for her endorsement and detailed review of my original manuscript, *Cat Care, Naturally,* my first book and foundation for this one, and for giving so much of her time and providing much valuable information. (Many thanks from Dr. Jean, as well, for her long-time friendship and for continuing to spread the principles of holistic medicine through her classes, books, and websites.)

Bill Inman, D.V.M., for his Veterinary Orthopedic Manipulation contribution, and Charles Loops, D.V.M., for his review of my original manuscript and useful input.

Special thanks to David Getoff and the Price-Pottenger Nutrition Foundation, Sally Fallon, and The Weston A. Price Foundation.

Jim McMullan for giving me the confidence to present this material to the world; and Leslie Rugg, whose belief in me helped make this book a reality.

Grace Freedson, my wonderful literary agent; my publisher, Quarry Books; my editor Rochelle Bourgault; and all of their team members.

My mother, Helene Yarnall, for teaching me to shoot for the stars; my daughter, Camilla, my son-in-law, Steven Forte, and my granddaughter, Gabrielle, for their love and support; Irene Kane and Phil Forte for all they do for our family.

Siegfried, Roy, and Lynette for their support through the years; Bill and Elizabeth Shatner, for their inspiration and friendship; Bob Weatherwax and Laddie, for sharing their animal training tips.

T.S. Wiley (Susie), author of *Lights Out and Sex, Lies, and Menopause*, as well as the creator of The Wiley Protocol. The antiaging advice she has generously provided keeps me going strong!

Special thanks to Marla Wilson for introducing me to The Wiley Protocol.

Many thanks to Carlton Lee for his friendship and all his work on the resources section of this book.

Special thanks from Dr. Jean to Dr. Michael Fox as a great friend and mentor, but most of all for his passion for helping animals; and to Steve Blake, D.V.M., for getting me started on the right foot in holistic medicine.

The Cat Fanciers' Association (CFA) all of our CFA judges; and Sandee and Dale Gilbert, our tireless CFA cat show veterans and my breeding partners in our sister cattery, Celestkats.

All of our cat clients and friends who have supported my work through the years, including the Tonkinese Breed Association, Tonkinese Breed Council, Tonks West, the Oriental Shorthair Breed Council, and the Cat Writers Association.

The entire eleven generations of Celestecats/Celestkats cats and kittens, for the love they have given unconditionally and the lessons they have taught us.

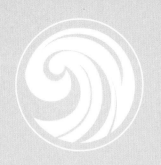

ABOUT
THE AUTHORS

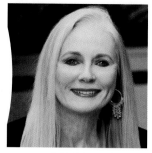

© 2009 Steven Silverstein

CELESTE YARNALL, PH.D.

Celeste Yarnall has lived a multifaceted life. You may remember her as a guest-starring actress on the classic *Star Trek* episode entitled "The Apple." Or perhaps as Elvis Presley's costar in *Live a Little, Love a Little*. You may even have seen her in the world of commercial real estate in Beverly Hills, California, where she owned and operated Celeste Yarnall and Associates Commercial Real Estate Services. Perhaps you knew that she managed screenwriters and sold several projects to major film studios.

Her lifetime love of cats and dogs led to the adoption of a collie puppy, a litter with Lassie 5, more collies and ultimately, Tonkinese and Oriental Shorthair cats. She quickly realized that there was much to be challenged in the world of traditional veterinary medicine, which led her to study clinical nutrition; in 1997, she was awarded a doctorate in Nutrition from Pacific Western University.

Her first book, *Cat Care Naturally*, was published in 1995. The updated paperback, *Natural Cat Care*, was published in 1998. Celeste is also the author of *Natural Dog Care*.

Between 1993 and 2009, Celeste and her breeding partners have bred and raised eleven generations of Tonkinese championship show cats on the basic holistic principals outlined in her books.

A lifetime interest in nutritional supplementation inspired Celeste to create a line of all-natural whole food supplements with holistic veterinarian Russell Swift, D.V.M. These formulas have been used for many years in her breeding program. In 2000, Celeste and Imelda Lopez-Casper formed Celestial Pets, whose products are available on their website and at a select group of retail stores. Ever conscious of trying to make the species-specific diet for cats easy to prepare, Celeste Yarnall Foods was born, incorporating naturally-raised meats, bones, and poultry prepared by their local butcher according to the partners' strict requirements and then flash frozen.

Celestial Pets offers a clinical nutrition consultation service, making available a host of products and services, including books, herbs, Chinese herbal medicine, homeopathics, homotoxicology, flower essences, and natural flea prevention. The company also provides life coaching on antiaging, weight loss, and holistic alternatives for people, too.

Today, Celeste relaxes by playing her concert grand pedal harp and dancing Argentine Tango! She loves to travel, especially to Italy, where she can practice her second language, Italian.

Visit www.celestialpets.com to see the Celestecats Tonkinese cats and kittens, the fresh raw food diet they are raised on, along with the Celestial Pets supplements and all the other good things currently going on at Celestial Pets. Check back often for information on new advances in veterinary medicine, holistic therapies, and new products we find that we think will be of interest to you.

Our goal is to be your source for information in the world of holistic health care for cats—and dogs. For more information call 818.707.6331 or email us at celestialpet@sbcglobal.net.

For more information on Celeste's filmography, visit www.celesteyarnall.com.

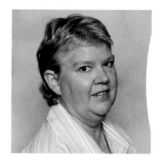

JEAN HOFVE, D.V.M.

Dr. Jean Hofve earned her Doctor of Veterinary Medicine at Colorado State University in Fort Collins, Colorado. In her third year of veterinary school, she was introduced to veterinary homeopathy by Christina Chambreau, D.V.M., and her life was never the same again.

Dr. Jean practiced holistic and conventional medicine in Denver, Colorado; and was the editor-in-chief of the *Journal of the American Holistic Veterinary Medical Association* from 2004 through 2007, when she retired. She has extensive training in homeopathy and homotoxicology, and in 1995 founded Spirit Essences, which remains the only veterinarian-formulated line of flower essences for animals.

Dr. Jean is internationally recognized for her expertise on holistic pet health, pet food, and nutrition. Her articles have appeared in *Animal Wellness*, *The Whole Dog Journal*, *The Whole Cat Journal*, *Cats*, *DogWorld*, *Journal of the Academy of Veterinary Homeopathy*, and *Journal of the American Holistic Veterinary Medical Association*. She worked for the Animal Protection Institute (API) as their Companion Animal Program Coordinator for two years, and she served as advisor to the Association of American Feed Control Officials, the standard-setting organization for pet food, on API's behalf. Her website, www.littlebigcat.com, is a respected source of information on feline holistic health, nutrition, and behavior.

Dr. Jean lives in Denver, Colorado, with four fabulous felines: Flynn, Puzzle, Sundance, and Spencer. She unwinds by playing the ukulele with a local band called the Blue Ukeladies (www.blueukeladies.com).

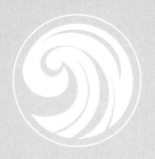

INDEX

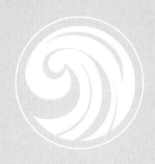

PHOTOGRAPER CREDITS

Diane Amble & Firenza Pini, 129

© Juniors Bildarchiv/agefotostock.com, 48; 64

Paul Bricknell/gettyimages.com, 88

Courtesy of Celestial Pets/www.celestialpets.com, 10; 30 (left); 56; 120; 151

Sharon DeCeuninck, 39; 84; 122

© Roberto della Vite/agefotostock.com, 81

Cathie Ernst, 80

www.fioriperlanima.com, 107 (top)

Fotolia.com, 16, 18; 21; 28; 52; 54; 60; 70; 92; 114; 119; 132; 145; 157

David Getoff, 11

Dr. Jean Hofve, 102 (top); 103 (top & second); 104 (second); 104 (bottom); 105 (bottom); 107 (bottom)

iStockphoto.com, 6; 14; 25; 26; 32; 36; 38; 42; 47; 50; 65; 69; 73; 78; 83; 91; 102 (middle & bottom); 103 (third & bottom); 104 (top & third); 105 (top, second & third); 106; 107 (second & third); 108; 110; 123; 124; 126; 136; 138; 143; 144; 156

Courtney Kahler, 22

Richard Katris/Chanon Photography, www.chanon. com, 5; 19; 24; 29; 34; 40; 66; 76; 77; 150

Carlton Lee, 53

Marc Liberts, 146

Linda & Carmen Martino, 30 (right); 31

Kevin Mootsey, 86; 111; 131; 135; 148

© David Muscroft/agefotosotck.com, 94

Denise Raupach, 100; 112; 115; 139, 140

© Marco Scataglini/agefotostock.com, 62

www.shutterstock.com, 141

© Frank Siteman/agefotostock.com, 20

Carl J. Widmer, 13